Ágnes Rosecker
Zoltán Bajory

Vaseline Injection, an Inadequate Method for Penile Augmentation

Ágnes Rosecker
Zoltán Bajory

Vaseline Injection, an Inadequate Method for Penile Augmentation

LAP LAMBERT Academic Publishing

Impressum / Imprint
Bibliografische Information der Deutschen Nationalbibliothek: Die Deutsche Nationalbibliothek verzeichnet diese Publikation in der Deutschen Nationalbibliografie; detaillierte bibliografische Daten sind im Internet über http://dnb.d-nb.de abrufbar.
Alle in diesem Buch genannten Marken und Produktnamen unterliegen warenzeichen-, marken- oder patentrechtlichem Schutz bzw. sind Warenzeichen oder eingetragene Warenzeichen der jeweiligen Inhaber. Die Wiedergabe von Marken, Produktnamen, Gebrauchsnamen, Handelsnamen, Warenbezeichnungen u.s.w. in diesem Werk berechtigt auch ohne besondere Kennzeichnung nicht zu der Annahme, dass solche Namen im Sinne der Warenzeichen- und Markenschutzgesetzgebung als frei zu betrachten wären und daher von jedermann benutzt werden dürften.

Bibliographic information published by the Deutsche Nationalbibliothek: The Deutsche Nationalbibliothek lists this publication in the Deutsche Nationalbibliografie; detailed bibliographic data are available in the Internet at http://dnb.d-nb.de.
Any brand names and product names mentioned in this book are subject to trademark, brand or patent protection and are trademarks or registered trademarks of their respective holders. The use of brand names, product names, common names, trade names, product descriptions etc. even without a particular marking in this works is in no way to be construed to mean that such names may be regarded as unrestricted in respect of trademark and brand protection legislation and could thus be used by anyone.

Coverbild / Cover image: www.ingimage.com

Verlag / Publisher:
LAP LAMBERT Academic Publishing
ist ein Imprint der / is a trademark of
OmniScriptum GmbH & Co. KG
Heinrich-Böcking-Str. 6-8, 66121 Saarbrücken, Deutschland / Germany
Email: info@lap-publishing.com

Herstellung: siehe letzte Seite /
Printed at: see last page
ISBN: 978-3-659-53295-5

Zugl. / Approved by: Szeged, University of Szeged, 2014

Copyright © 2014 OmniScriptum GmbH & Co. KG
Alle Rechte vorbehalten. / All rights reserved. Saarbrücken 2014

Acknowledgements

First and foremost I wish to express my gratitude to Prof. Dr. László Pajor and to my urological training tutor Dr. Olivér Pintér for having been given the opportunity and for the ongoing support in my vocational training.

I am particularly grateful to my supervisor, Dr. Zoltán Bajory for his constant help and inspiration.

I would like to offer my special thanks for his assistance in doing the statistics to Károly Acsai.

And I am obliged to all my colleagues for their support in everyday work and in the treatment of patients alike.

I thank almighty to my family, without whom I would have never gone this far.

I wish to thank various people for their contribution to this project: to Dr. Antal Kökényesi pi Lieutenant General, National Commander in Chief, who made it possible to carry out our survey, as well as to the commanders of the prisons: Tibor Frank pi Brigadier Senior Counsellor (Budapest Penitentiary and Prison), László Biczó pi Brigadier General (Márianosztra Prison), Tamás Rózsahegyi pi Lieutenant Colonel (Sátoraljaújhely Prison), Dr. Zoltán Pantali pi Brigadier General, Senior Counsellor (Sopronkőhida Prison), Dr. Pál Kiszely pi Brigadier General, Senior Counsellor (Szeged Prison), Gyula Vatai pi. Colonel. (Váci Prison). I would also like to extend my grateful thanks to the prison employees, who helped our work.

Table of Contents

Table of Contents — 2
- *List of Figures* — 3
- *List of Tables* — 4

Introduction — 5
- *Historical Overview* — 5
- *The Normal Penis Size and the Need for Augmentation* — 6
- *The Classification of Foreign Materials Inserted into the Penis* — 7
- *Foreign Bodies Inserted into the Urethra* — 7
- *Strangulation* — 9
- *Intim Piercings* — 11
- *Materials Inserted Under the Skin of the Penis* — 12
- *Penile Nodules* — 12
- *Penis Enlargement, Vaseline and Other Materials* — 15
- *Penile Augmentation with Allograft and Xenograft Materials* — 15
- *Hyaluronic Acid* — 16
- *Methacrylate Injection* — 17
- *Other Fillers* — 17
- *Vaseline* — 18
- *Treatment* — 19
- *The Epidemiology of Vaseline in and outside Prisons in Hungary* — 21
- *Non-Invasive Methods of Penis Lengthening* — 21
- *Vacuum Device* — 21
- *Penile Traction Therapy* — 21
- *Invasive Procedures to Increase the Penis* — 22
- *Extending with Rib Cartilage* — 22
- *Phalloplasty Augmentation with Bilateral Saphena Grafts* — 22
- *Suprapubic Dermatolipectomy with Liposuction* — 23
- *Penile Suspensory Ligament Division* — 23

The Aim of the Thesis — 23

Methods — 24
- *Our Cohort* — 24
- *Questionnaire Survey in Prisons* — 28
- *Statistical Analysis* — 29

Results — 30
- *Demographic Data* — 30
- *The Results of the Questionnaire Survey* — 32

Discussion — 40

Summary of New Scientific Results — 43

List of Figures

Figure 1 A: Penis incarcerated by an iron ring **B:** Removal with metal saw **C:** Penis after the removal **D:** Control examination, after one week.

Figure 2 Piercing Prince Albert

Figure 3 The patient has inserted Vaseline and penile nodules under the skin of the penis

Figure 4 The removed nodules

Figure 5 After the operation

Figure 6 The pedicle island flap is pulled up to the dorsal surface of the penis through a subcutaneous tunnel.

Figure 7 The penile skin defect is replaced.

Figure 8 The bare skinned penis is placed in a tunnel under the tunica dartos of the scrotum.

Figure 9 The scrotal-skin flap is transluminated. The anterior scrotal branches of the deep external pudendal artery and the posterior scrotal branches of the internal pudendal artery are visualized.

Figure 11 Questionnaire

Figure 12 15.7% (N=299) of the responders, admitted that they had injected Vaseline into their penis

Figure 13 The effect of injecting Vaseline on sexual life. A) Those, who did not have Vaseline injected, B) Vaseline adopters.

Figure 14 Penile abnormalities in patients with complications of Vaseline self-injection

Figure 15 22.4% of the Vaseline users regretted the self-injection; however, the rate who had complications was 53%; 72.4%, who regretted the Vaseline self-injection would undergo a reconstructive surgery to remove Vaseline

Figure 16 Relationship between the mean amounts of Vaseline injected and mean duration of hospitalization in Groups A-C

Figure 17 A: The testicles are covered by the femoral transposition flaps **B:** Three months postoperatively; the femoral transposition flaps have slightly shrunk, but the patient experienced only discomfort

List of Tables

Table 1 A The proportion of the Hungarian convicts categorized
Table 1 B The inmates' education by the length of their sentence
Table 1 C The inmates' marital status
Table 2 The proportion of the convicts categorized by the length of their sentence
Table 3 Different groups who recommended Vaseline self-injection to the respondent subjects
Table 4 Different types of procedures by groups
Table 5 Descriptive statistics of patients in Group A-C

Introduction

Historical Overview

Since time immemorial, men experiment with increasing the size of their penis. The penis is the symbol of masculinity, fertility and power (Kadouch et al., 2012), so no wonder that people have tried to extend it in various ways. In some subcultures the habit of self-harm of the penis for augmentation is widespread today, as well. Inserted foreign bodies in the penis have been known for long in several cultures. The first archaeological finds, that suggest surgical intervention to ornament the penis, are from the late Palaeolithic age (12 700 years) (Angulo et al., 2011). The first written reference to enhance sexual pleasure and to increase the size of the penis was in the Kama Sutra. Small round objects were placed under the skin of the penis, or were decorated on it. (Stankov et al., 2009) Drilling through penis was widespread with the Romans, also. They put wood, metal and bone into it (Józsa, 2011).

The other interventions of sexuality, which were not for enhancing, but inhibitory processes, are also as old as mankind. However, the interventions impeding erection were carried out mostly by doctors. The infibulation was a procedure in which the foreskin was pulled down to the end of the penis, holes were punched into it in many places, then a metal wire was pulled in it after the scarring, and the ends were colligated. These chastity belts were pin or ring-shaped and their bearer could get rid of it only with medical help. The first written record comes from the Roman Aulus Cornelius Celsus 25 B.C. In ancient times young singer boys had it to slow sexual maturation so that their voice didn't mutate, and it was common among the harp artists and actors, who wore the ring as jewellery hanging out from their garment. Later, from the eighteenth to the beginning of the twentieth century it served to prevent masturbation and it was connected with the misbelief of masturbation causing epilepsy. The infibulation was widespread in Germany and in the U.S. in the nineteenth century, and major experts also believed in its efficiency (Schultheiss et al., 2003).

The first strangulation case was published by Gauthier in 1775. Since then, many cases are known where the penis was damaged this way (Gauthier, 1755).

It was about one and a half thousand years ago when the habit of placing tiny jades or metals under the skin of the penis spread from Indochina. The mainly in Slavic and Asian cultures prevalent implants to increase sexuality have already reached the western cultures. The method was probably spread out by the soldiers in World War II, although it is disputed by some authors (Stankov et al., 2009).

The Vaseline has been being used for penile augmentation or thickening for more than 100 years. The petroleum jelly was first applied by a Viennese surgeon Robert Gersuny after a castration in 1899 to replace a young boy's testicles, as he lost both of them due to tuberculosis (Glicenstein, 2007).

The Normal Penis Size and the Need for Augmentation

Many men have a wrong idea about the normal penis size, they are worried that their penis is not big enough and they cannot satisfy their partner. The false body image that the penis is smaller than the normal size is a form of small penis syndrome, which is a type of psychosis, as professionals call it, dysmorphophobia or body dysmorphic disorder. The dysmorphophobia can lead to serious psychiatric disorders, erectile dysfunction or social problems (Wylie and Eardley, 2007). This incorrect perception of the size of the penis can develop in childhood. The patients see their penis smaller in comparison to their peers. This complex is later increased by pornography and the Internet, as well. In fact, what is the normal penis size? A few studies have dealt with the measurement of the penis, but the opinions differ in the measurement technique. Mondaini and colleagues did not measure the erect penis, only in the form of the flaccid and the stretched one. (Mondaini et al., 2002). In 1996, Wessels et al compared the penis measurement techniques in their study. They measured the length of the penis from the pubo-penile skin junction to the meatus. They measured the flaccid, the stretched and the erectile penis, as well. The average length of flaccid one was 8.8 cm, the stretched one was 12.4 cm and the erected one was 12.8 cm. Penis extender surgery is not recommended over flaccid 4 cm and stretched or erected over 7.5 cm (Wessel et al., 1996). Based on several studies according to Wylie and Eardley the average stretched size is between 12-13 cm and the erect length is between 14 and 16 cm. The mean girth is 9-10 cm when flaccid and 12-13 when erected (Wylie and Eardley, 2007).

The treatment can be conservative or surgical. Dysmorphophby always must be separated from micropenis, when the penis is really small. The non-surgical treatment option is the drug therapy like SSRI and anxiolytics for the patients. The testosterone therapy is recommended only in cases of real micropenis (Wylie and Eardley, 2007). The conservative therapy can be education, self-awareness and psychotherapy or physical treatment. The physical treatment uses vacuum devices, penile extenders and traction devices, penoscrotal and penile rings. (Aghamir et al., 2006, Oderda and Gontero, 2011). These methods are not very effective.

The length of the penis can be increased by pubopelvic liposuction, suspensory ligament dissection and skin flap construction. The thickening of the penis is possible by injecting various substances, such as autologous fat, hyaluronic acid and silicone (Kang et al., 2012). There are men with normal sized penis who wish enlargement surgery. With these surgeries length can be extended by 1-2 cm and the thickness by 2.5 cm in average. The surgeries may also have a number of complications, penile deformity, penile instability, paradoxical penile shortening, scarring, the development of granule, the migration of the injected material and sexual dysfunction (Vardi et al., 2008).

The Classification of Foreign Materials Inserted into the Penis

The foreign substances placed into the penis with the intention of enhancing sexual performance can be divided into four groups, cases of strangulation, objects shoved into the urethra for the purpose of stiffening and objects or liquid implanted under the skin of the penis to thicken it, or for aesthetic aspects.

The frequency of self-injuries of the penis is currently increasing in certain cultures. Practitioners are often faced with complications caused by metals, plastics or semi liquids inserted into the penis. The use of penile nodules and petroleum jelly is mainly widespread in Asia and Eastern Europe, particularly in prisons, whereas body piercing is rather fashionable in Western cultures.

The aim of using such penile foreign bodies may be the enhancing of sexual performance, to prolong an erection, sexual curiosity, to achieve erotic or auto-erotic effects, masturbation, contraception or to prevent enuresis (Stankov et al., 2009; van Ophoven and de Kernion, 2000).

Foreign Bodies Inserted into the Urethra

Various objects have been inserted into the urethra for different reasons, like maintaining the erection, sexual curiosity, masturbation and contraception purposes, or to prevent enuresis (van Ophoven et al., 2000). The convicts in prisons insert objects into their penis in the hope of some medical treatment outside the prison (Mastromichalis et al., 2011). Misinformed children by the Internet experiment (Sinopidis et al., 2012). The patients' age is different, they may be mentally retarded or suffering from mental illness, as well. The foreign bodies known to have been applied for this purpose include glass rods, hooks, knitting needles, pins, pencils, ball pens, pen holders, hairpins, matches, electric wires, vine branches, parts of rubber rings, necklaces, forks, forceps, straws, screws, pistachio shells, razor blades, a toothbrush, an Allen key, drill bits, eye droppers, pacifiers, etc. (van Ophoven and de Kernion, 2000; Walsh and Moustafa, 2000; Molnár and Szőke, 1973; Sukkarieh et al., 2004; Mitterberger et al., 2009; Brison et al., 2006; Sinopidis et al., 2012). Extreme cases of a 45 cm headless snake (van Ophoven and de Kernion, 2000) and broken mirror have also been reported (Hwang et al., 2010). The meatus has already been clogged up with chewing gum, dropped in candle wax, inserted beans for contraceptive purpose. (van Ophoven et al., 2000; Molnár et al., 1973). Not only rigid objects can be inserted into the urethra, but some liquid, as well (usually water) for autoerotic purposes, thereby augmenting it; the procedure is called "urethral sounding" (Breyer and Shindel 2012). Those who practice "urethral sounding" belong to the high-risk groups (promiscuity), they more often suffer from venereal disease (Rinard et al., 2010). Kokkonouzis et al reported an unusual case; a Bulgarian immigrant filled paraffin in his urethra and lengthened it with a string. Although he deformed his penis significantly he refused any treatment (Kokkonouzis et al., 2008).

Foreign materials inserted into the urethra can give rise to mechanical irritation, inflammation, urethral discharge, ascending urinary tract infections, haematuria, dysuria, painful erections and sepsis or uraemia. The long-term consequences may include urethral stricture, diverticulum, incontinence or erectile dysfunction (Stankov et al., 2009; van Ophoven et al., 2000; Walsh et al., 2000; Sukkarieh et al., 2004; Mastromichelis et al., 2011; Sinopidis et al., 2012). To set up a diagnosis the careful medical history record is essential. The patients are often embarrassed by their action, or they are mentally retarded, so a medical history cannot be obtained. If the first health worker has no suspicion of a foreign body in the urethra, it can be easily pushed up to the bladder by bladder catheterization causing further complications or the appropriate treatment can be delayed due to the late diagnosis. In some cases radiographic visible imaging techniques can help. With this treatment it is important to remove the foreign object as soon as possible, using cystoscopy or open surgery, which can depend on the size and the material of the object and on the chance of causing a further effect of the injury. The treatment is mainly endoscopic. Antibiotic therapy is recommended in all cases (Sukkarieh et al., 2004). If the patient can drain the bladder, there is no need to insert a catheter (Walsh et al., 2000).

Strangulation

Various items are pulled on the penis that can cause strangulation. They pull metal rings, wedding rings, iron sleeves, nuts, pipes, bearings, bicycle parts, all kinds of bottles, PET bottles, tools, hair or rubber bands, on their penis (van Ophoven and de Kernion, 2000; Ivanovski et al., 2007, Pannek and Martin, 2003). In cases of strangulation the patients often turn to a doctor because they cannot remove the trapped objects from their penis. The success of the treatment depends on the occlusion device, on the removal device and on the elapsed time. Unfortunately, patients often wait days, months, or years for seeing the doctor, whereas over 72 hours good result cannot be expected. The patients' age varies between wide limits. Their usual aim is to achieve an erotic and autoerotic effect, or the extension of their erection (Silberstein et al., 2008). With young children the aim can be the prevention of enuresis, as well (van Ophoven and de Kernion, 2000).

These objects can be made of metal or non-metal material. The non-metallic objects can cause more serious injuries, but their removal is easier. The non-metal objects are more flexible, therefore the greater pressure effect on the penis can cause more damage (Silberstein et al., 2008; Mooreville et al., 2011). Objects pulled onto or wound round the penis can cause mechanical damage. The clamping of the penis causes venous stasis or blockage. As a result of venous stasis, the penis swells and the lymph vessels and arteries may then be blocked, with the consequence of ischaemia or infarction. After several hours, necrosis and gangrene may develop. In some cases, not only the penis, but also the scrotum is ligated (Silberstein et al., 2008). Bhat et al. divided the injuries into 5 groups.

Group 1: oedema in the distal area.
Group 2: the injury of the skin and the corpus spongiosum, reduced sensation
Group 3: the injury of the skin and the urethra, loss of distal penile sensation
Group 4: the separation of the corpus spongiosum, the constriction of the urethral fistula and the corpus cavernosum and the loss of distal penile sensation
Group 5: gangrene, necrosis, distal or total amputation of the penis (Bhat el al., 1991)
Whereas Silberstein et al. simplified the grouping classifying the injuries as low-grade or high-grade (Silberstein et al., 2008).
The most important task is to remove the foreign body, which can involve serious technical difficulties in case of metals. The treatment and the removal of the device

depend on the way and the time of the ram, the patient's cooperation and on the doctor's available devices. The degree of vascular injury can be concluded with Colour Doppler ultrasonography after the performed removal of the object. The device causing the tourniquet should be removed as quickly as possible, so as not to cause further injury. Anaesthesia is sometimes needed, as well. The removing of metal objects may require metal cutting devices. Bolt cutters, electric saws, diamond headed drills, dental drills can be used (Kang et al., 2002; Lamba et al., 2012; Kelemen et al., 2005; Király et al., 2007) (figure 1.). To avoid further injury it is worth to place a protecting metal object between the clamping device and the penis, which can be a laryngoscope cap (Peay et al., 2009), as well and cooling is advisable during the process.

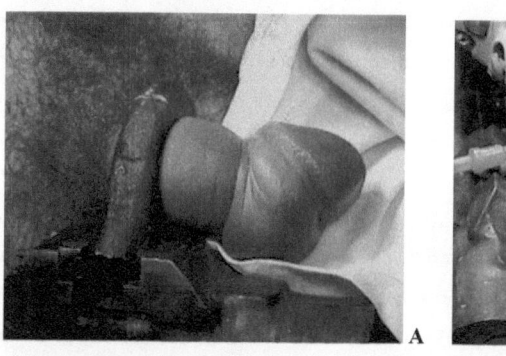
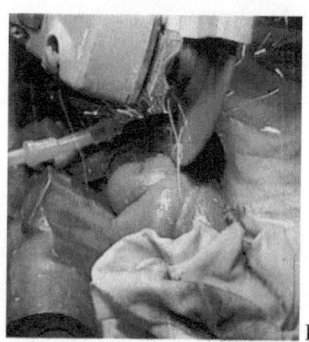
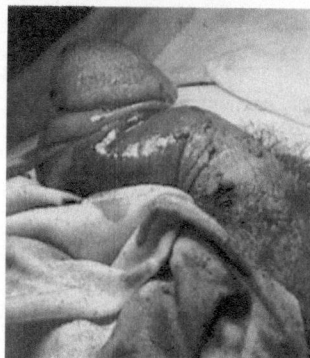
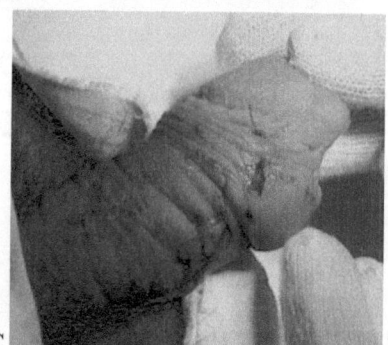

Figure 1 A: *Penis incarcerated by an iron ring* **B:** *Removal with metal saw*
C: *Penis after the removal* **D:** *Control examination one week later*

Non-invasive removal techniques are also known. Under the clamp object a thread can be led and the object can be removed from the penis with its help (String techniques) (Noh et al., 2004). The stagnant blood or oedema can be reduced with pressure on the glans, or drained with the help of puncture (Dundee-technique) (Pastides et al., 2011), thus the diameter of the penis decreases and the clamp can be pulled off. The two techniques can be combined. The enhanced version is the pseudo-pulley technique; the oedema can be drained with the help of a needle, and a tourniquet placed on previously prevents the re-formation of the oedema. Four needle guide wires should be placed under the metal bearing. The tourniquet should be removed, the penis should be lubricated and with the help of the needle guide wire the bearing should be pulled off (Katz et al., 2012). In rare cases, the damage is so severe that the penis cannot be saved and it must be amputated (Ivanovski et al., 2007, Silberstein et al., 2008). After the removal of the clamping objects the development of other infections is to be prevented, so patients should receive tetanus and antibiotic prophylaxis. The analysis of the urine and microbiological culturing is essential. Urinary diversion is needed if the patient is unable to urinate; in this case epicystostoma puncture is recommended (Silberstein et al., 2008).

Intim Piercings

The spread of tattoo and body piercing has been rapidly increasing in Western societies over the last 20 years; however, the appropriate professional background is far below the hygienic requirements. The most common type of jewellery is the Prince Albert piercing, which is a ring pierced on the ventral side of the penis and urethra, as well. The Ampallang piercing drills through the glands and the urethra across, while the Apadravya does it lengthwise touching the urethra, as well. The less popular Frenum is put in the frenulum, while the Dyode drills through the coronaries (Nelius et al. 2011, Anderson et al. 2003).

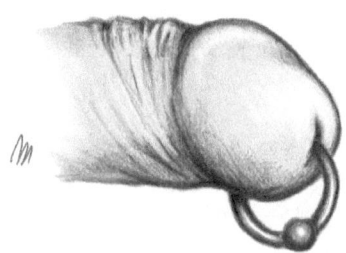

Figure 2 *Prince Albert piercing*

Objects used in modern piercing are made of surgical steel or titanium. Unfortunately, the piercing objects worn by men perforate not only the glans, but additionally the urethra, which can result in serious complications and can also change the urinary flow. The piercings are usually implanted in specialized parlours, where the health standards are mostly ensured, but complications may still develop. To insert the piercing is easy: the location is drawn on the skin, which is disinfected, and with a pair of pliers the skin is pinched, then it is punctured with an indwelling cannula, and finally the piercing is put in (Anderson et al., 2003).

Several surveys identified demographic characteristics, motivations and health problems among males who had body piercing. The respondents were typically from the younger age group, and the main motivations proved to be sexual stimulation, experimentation and fashion (Rinard et al. 2010, Anderson et al., 2003, Caliendo 2005, Armstrong et al., 2006, and Skegg et al., 2005). Some publications explain the body piercing with the psychosocial behaviour of the patients. The risk taker is typical of these people (Holbrook et al., 2012, Gold et al., 2005, Ekelius et al., 2005 and Carroll et al., 2002).

The complications include STDs like condyloma acuminate and Chlamydia infection. Further complications can be: molluscum contagiosum, bleeding, inflammation, endocarditis, Fournier gangrene, allergic reactions, urethral stricture, fistulas, scars, keloids, paraphimosis, priapism, squamous cell carcinoma and injuries suffered by the partners. (Schultheiss et al. 2003, Gold et al., 2005, Carroll et al., 2002, Skegg et al., 2007, Blake-James et al., 2002, Gokhale et al., 2001, Scholten 2005, Edlin et al., 2010, Hounsfield and Davies 2008, Kaatz et al., 2008). Patients seek for medical advice only in severe cases; however the removal of the body jewellery itself could solve their problems. The prevention of complications caused by piercing should be the education of patients and the provision of professional background in the parlours.

Materials Inserted Under the Skin of the Penis
Penile Nodules

Nowadays in Asia, Eastern Europe, Argentina and Russia, small balls are inserted under the skin of the penis. The method is particularly popular among prisoners in Indonesia, Thai and Russian prisons, Israel (Russian immigrants), among the people of the Yakuza in Japan and in South California among the Hispanic inmates (Stankov et al., 2009; van Ophoven and Kernion 2000; Griffith and Horovitz 2012). The aim of the insertion of balls is to enhance the partner's sexual pleasure. Especially the female partner's joy is wished to be enhanced and it is not spread among homosexuals. The balls are polished of broken glass or plastic to the appropriate size. They can be made of ivory, precious stone, stone and gold, as well. They have different names such as Bolitas (the Philippines), Chagan balls (Korea), fang muk or Tancho (Thailand) sputnik (Russia) (Stankov and Ivanovski, 2009, Griffith and Horovitz, 2012). The number and the size of inserted balls can be different; they are usually 1 cm in diameter. Mostly 2-4, but sometimes even 10 pieces are inserted. The balls are placed underneath the penis skin so, that the first marks are engraved with a sharp object and through the small hole the polished plastic balls (e.g. made of a toothbrush handle) are placed in, and with using a stick or ball-point pen, they are pushed up in the tissues under the skin (Stankov and Ivanovski, 2009). Gürdal and colleagues reported a case, where stones were found under the patient's penile skin. They were inserted by a doctor in Saudi Arabia for penis enlargement. Although the stones did not cause any complications to the patient, the cosmetic result was unacceptable. The patient did not consent to the treatment (Gürdal et al., 2002).

Complications often develop. If they do not cause a problem, the wearer rarely turns to a doctor. Many times the patients remove the bullets themselves. The complications can be mostly bleedings, inflammation, and formation of a granuloma, ulceration, abscess, or a bruise in the partner's vagina. Some people inject Vaseline beside the balls into their penis for the purpose of magnification. The treatment consists of surgical removal of the bullets and conservative local treatment, which usually results a complete recovery. (Hsu 2004; Djajakusumat and Meheus, 2000; Cohen and Kim, 1982; Fischer et al., 2010; Hudak et al., 2012; Lim et al., 1986; Levy et al., 2008; Hull and Budiharsana, 2001; Jaiswal, 1992; Silberstein et al., 2008).

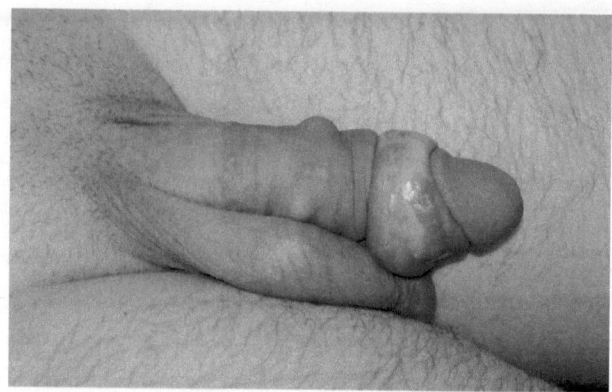

Figure 3 *The patient has inserted Vaseline and penile nodules under the skin of the penis*

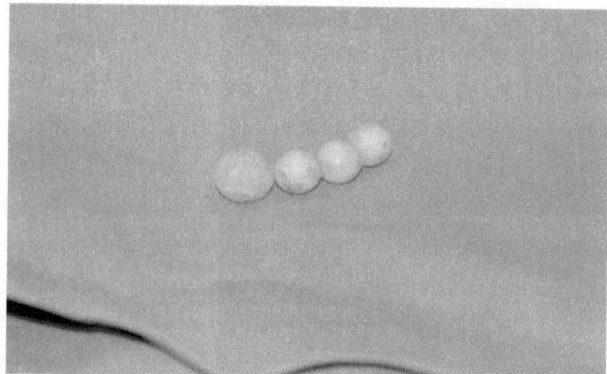

Figure 4 *The removed nodules*

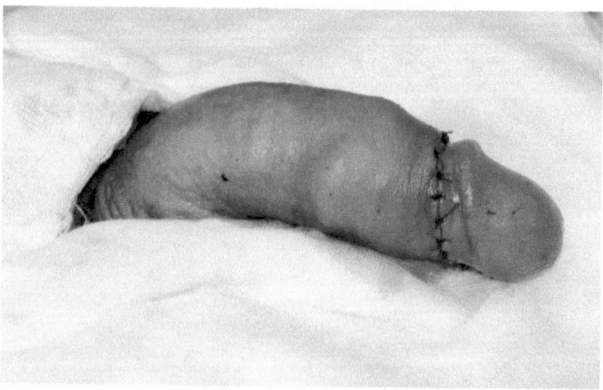

Figure 5 *After the operation*

Penis Enlargement, Vaseline and Other Materials

Liquid or semi-liquid material is injected under the skin of the penis for the sake of augmentation. Such materials are petroleum jelly, silicone, paraffin, formalin, alcohol, mineral oil, metallic mercury, transmission fluid, autologous fat and methacrylate (Torricelli et al., 2012; Kang et al., 2012).

Kadouch et al. distinguished 3 groups of liquid substances.

1: Absorbing or short-acting agents. They have an impact in a few months. These include collagen and hyaluronic acid.

2: Semipermanent or medium acting fillers. Their effect lasts for 6-12 months. These materials are the hyaluronic acid and the polyvinyl alcohol.

3: Permanent or long term fillers. They cause permanent damage. These are the silicone oil and 4% polyalkylimid (Kadouch et al., 2012).

Penile Augmentation with Allograft and Xenograft Materials

Free autologous fat graft can be used to make up tissue. Trockman at al. draw attention to the complications of penis thickening by autologous fat injection; it can cause inflammation, fibrosis, cyst formation and ecchymosis. The treatment of complications is usually surgical (Trockman et al., 1994). Kang et al. considered the method safe, there were hardly any complications. They followed 52 patients for more than 6 months. The aesthetic and functional results were satisfactory. The average initial thickness of the patients' penis was less than 7.4 cm. The fat was sucked down from the subcutaneous areas in the abdomen and thighs. The cleaned fat was injected right under the skin of the penis. The amount of the injected fat was between 25-49 ml. The obtained average thickness of the penis after the procedure was 9.31 cm (Kang et al., 2012).

In 2006 Perovic et al. followed 84 patients who had autologous tissue implant using biodegradable scaffolds for penis augmentation. They obtained fibroblasts by biopsy from the skin of the scrotum. They purified the cells; put them into tissue culture for at least 3 weeks. The tissue culture was put on dry polydactyl glycolic acid scaffold implant. The scaffold was placed between the dartos and Buck's fascia. 80% of the patients were satisfied with the achieved results; an average of 3.15 cm increase in the thickness of the penis. The complication rate was low (Perovic et al., 2006).

Solomon and colleagues reported a great number of complications with the use of allograft. The cellular dermal matrix is used by plastic surgeons for tissue deficits primarily in breast reconstruction surgery. This technique may be used for the thickening of the penis, as well. The allograft is laid on the Buck's fascia. The graft may come from a living donor or a cadaver. Three types of grafts were compared, but the complications occurred equally with grafts of different materials. They followed their patients for an average of 11.25 months. In 42% of the incidences infection and 6.4% total graft loss occurred. Because of the complications it's a pretty controversial method for penis thickening (Solomon et al., 2013).

Bruno and colleagues reported penis enlargement in connection with two cases of patients who lost skin because of necrosis. They made V-Y plastics AlloDermet (allograft dermal matrix) for penis enlargement and postoperative dorsal skin necrosis developed. They identified the cause of necrosis and it was mainly because of the damaged blood vessels by AlloDerm. The penile skin and prepucium is supplied by the inferior external pudendal superficial artery branches, which run bilaterally on the dorsal penile shaft. When these blood vessels get damaged, severe wound healing disturbances occur and the reconstruction is not easy. The treatment was combined with conservative wound care and they tried to preserve the remaining viable tissue with debridment as much as possible. The lack was made up by skin graft. The achieved cosmetic result was good (Bruno et al.. 2007).

Alei et al. used xenografts and porcine dermal acellular graft for penis thickening. They did not have major complications and they achieved approximately 3 cm thickening (Alei et al., 2012).

Hyaluronic Acid

Hyaluronic acid is used for the augmentation of the glans. The hyaluronic acid is injected directly in the glans, which is called the "mushroom technique". The technology comes from Asia. First Professor Sito applied it with bovine collagen. The hyaluronic is more bio-compatible than bovine collagen. 1-2 ml was injected from the sulcus coronary to the glans superficially every 2 months. Anaesthetic lidocaine / prilocaine cream was used to reduce pain. The complications were little; a small amount of bleeding and pain might occur. The patients were satisfied with the results. The glans increased of more than half inches in diameter (Micheels et al., 2012; Kim et al., 2003; Moon et al., 2003).

Methacrylate Injection

Torricelli et al reported a case, where methacrylate was injected into the penis for augmentation. The patient had his penis injected with methacrylate two years earlier in another private clinic. The patient was dissatisfied because the paste in his penis caused erection, aesthetic problems and pain. Torricelli et al. performed a reconstructive surgery, where the skin was removed along with the foreign substance and was replaced by a flap. The histology findings of the removed skin showed fibrosis and foreign body granuloma with amorphous material (Torricelli et al., 2013).

Sao Paulo Salles at al. treated their patients in their medical centre for polymethacrylat damage, among which there were patients who had had penis enlargement before. The polymethacrylat was suspended in purified bovine collagen or hyaluronic acid. The patients had complications like necrosis, granuloma formation, chronic inflammatory reaction and infection. If the material is injected too deeply into the arteries or veins, embolization may occur. Salles points out that neither the incidence nor the prevalence of the cases is known. There are no standardized treatment guidelines or principles either; they need to be developed (Salles et al., 2008).

Shaeer and Shaeer reported a case, where polyacrylamide gel was used for the patient's penis enlargement and years later complications developed. The patient had granuloma formation and migration of the foreign material under the skin. The affected skin was separated, which was not easy because the mass stuck to the Buck's fascia, the corpus cavernosums and corpus spongiosum in some places. The material was carefully separated while taking care of the neurovascular bundle. Then the wound was closed with the rest of the penis skin in two layers. As a result, histology showed chronic inflammation and fibrosis (Shaeer and Shaeer, 2009).

Other Fillers

Manny et al. in their article write about immigrant to the U.S. from Laos, who injected suspense called "Super Extenze". This illegal substance contained mineral oil and vitamin E (Manny et al. 2011).

Silicone

Attempts have been made for penis augmentation with silicone for a long time (Arthaud, 1973; Narins and Beer, 2006). The penis augmentation with silicone causes paraffinoma and the same complications as Vaseline does (Shamsodini et al., 2012; Silberstein et al., 2008).

Kadouch et al. presented 6 of their cases, where the patients appeared several weeks after the action due to severe complications. They injected fluid (silicone oil, polyalkylimide) into their penis or scrotum to enlarge their penis. The procedure was performed by a plastic surgeon or urologist several times in different countries. On the spot of the intervention, inflammation developed and the patients had high fever. In all cases they performed surgery and applied a broad spectrum antibiotic treatment. The authors considered the only possible solution to remove the inflamed tissue. They did not recommend the filling of genitals with fluids from aesthetic reasons (Kadouch et al., 2012). The silicone filling process for penis augmentation is not safe either. A number of adverse reactions were reported. In a case the biopsy histology record reported verucosus SCC, and after the histological processing of the removed material it turned out that it was a severe inflammation (Magrill et al., 2008). Solving the damage caused by silicone the same surgical techniques are known as for Vaseline (Yacobi et al., 2007).

Vaseline

The self-injection of Vaseline is still a widely used method for penis thickening in Eastern Europe and Asia, especially among ex-convict men. It occurs sporadically in other parts of the world, due to the immigrants, such as Portugal (Ukrainian immigrants) (Santos et al., 2003), and Wisconsin Hmong (an Asian ethnic group) (Zickerman and Ratanawong, 2007).

The most serious complication of penis harming process is maybe the self-injection of Vaseline. The heated Vaseline (10-80 ml) is injected under the skin of the penis, mostly in poor sanitary conditions by layman inexperienced in health care. The Vaseline is massaged evenly over the skin of the penis and the patient is laid prone for a day so that the Vaseline cannot flow off the foreskin, as it would cause severe stenosis. The necessary material and equipment (needles, syringes and Vaseline) are not expensive and are easily accessible for prisoners, as well. Most often untrained persons perform the procedure paying no attention to sterility, and the hygiene requirements are usually ignored. Based on these facts, it is not surprising that the rate of complications is high and severe cases are not uncommon either. The fatty substances injected into the penis (Vaseline, paraffin oil, silicone) result granulomatous foreign body reaction in the damaged tissue. The consequences of foreign body reaction can be the acute inflammation and after a few months chronic inflammation, fibrosis and microcirculatory disturbances occur in the affected skin. Histologically the damage is a sclerosing lipogranuloma (Santos et al., 2003; Steffens et al., 2000; Cohen et al., 2001; Kelemen et al., 2006; Carlson, 1968; Nakamura et al., 1985; Imbert et al., 2010; Soyer et al; 1988). The early reaction is that the penis swells; the skin becomes red, hot and painful. The patients can have fever then ulcers and abscesses and fistulas may also develop. After the acute symptoms, complications may develop such as phimosis, urinating difficulty, scarring, chronic ulcers, skin necrosis, gangrene and erectile dysfunction (Santos et al., 2003; Carlson, 1968). The complications rarely evolve immediately, but after months or years of the self-injection of Vaseline. It is made by the patients to emphasize their masculinity, but instead of the desired effect often complications ensue. Patients often cannot tell what they did when they see the doctor so the diagnosis is late or unnecessary imaging tests are made. A Laotian immigrant was treated with steroids, as the lesion lichen sclerosus et atrophicus was diagnosed (Manny et al., 2011). As for the diagnosis, primarily a sexual disease (lymphogranuloma venerum), tuberculosis, or tumour must be distinguished (Sejben et al., 2012; Ko et al., 2004). As the process is illegal and causes unpleasant situations or complications and the reconstructive surgery is expensive, they try to hide both the proceedings and the complications. The population in question rarely seeks for help; therefore there are no adequate literature data about the incidence and the frequency of complications concerning Vaseline self-injection. There are only a few publications in the literature, which are mostly case reports focusing on the surgical procedures and complications (Tóth et al., 1984; May and Pickering, 1956; Wiwanitkit, 2004; Pehlivanov et al., 2008; Al-Ansari et al., 2010 ; Karakan et al., 2012; Torricelli et al., 2013). The treatment is surgical, as conservative treatment is not a permanent solution.

Treatment

Akkus et al. in a case tried intralesional steroid injections and warm bath as the patient refused the surgery. The therapy was not successful (Akkus et al., 2006, Rosenberg et al., 2007).

The removing of Vaseline is only possible together with the affected skin. In all the cases early surgical reconstruction resulted healing. The damaged areas should be cut out and a plastic replacement is needed (Rosenberg et al., 2007, Nyirády et al., 2008; Bayraktar and Basar, 2012). Different surgical techniques were also described, ranging from simple excision of the granuloma to a difficult two-stage surgery when the penis was implanted into the scrotum. The skin coverage techniques were the scrotal flaps, inguinal flaps, free flaps, or split-thickness skin grafts (Santucci et al., 2000).

Lee et al. dealt with the branches of the vessels nourishing the scrotal skin, but they did not mention the precise technique for the identification of the scrotal vascularity (Lee et al., 1994).

Steffens et al. emphasize the radical removal of the Vaseline granuloma and at the same time the organ-sparing surgery, as well. Five cases were operated; the patients were Russian immigrants with Vaseline granulomas. A one-stage operation was carried out with mesh-graft transplantation to replace excised defects. In the case of larger skin deficits a two-stage surgery was made. The naked penis was placed under the skin of the scrotum for three months. The tension of the penile skin was released by dorsal slit incision. The skin defects of the penis were covered with meshed grafts (Steffens et al., 2000).

The two-staged surgical technique of the scrotal tunnel flap: the damaged skin and the subcutaneous tissue should be removed to the Buck's fascia. A vertical incision is made at the down part of the scrotum and a subcutanous scrotal tunnel should be developped. The subcoronal penile skin must be fixed to the edges of the distal scrotal tunnel. The incision at the base of the penis should be closed with interrupted suture. Then in 3 months the penis should be taken out by linear incision or W-shaped flaps or Z-plasty (Parnitvidikun, 2007).

The restoration of the skin can be carried out by bilateral scrotal flaps, as well (Santucci et al., 2000; Jung et al., 2012).The damaged skin should be removed, but the neurovascular bundle and the Buck's fascia must be preserved. Then the flaps should be lifted with the Dartos fascia. To ensure the bleeding control is very important. Only a Z-plastic is made in the ventral suture line and a new penoscrotal junction should be created. Thus the penile shaft will look shorter (Jindarak et al., 2005). Shin and colleagues developed a new technique for replacing the penile skin: the T-style anastomosis with bilateral scrotal flaps. The skin affected by paraffin should be entirely removed. The bilateral scrotal flaps are dorsally-stitched together to the corona glandis. The shaft skin is also replaced from the skin of the scrotum ventrally. An inverted Vshaped incision is made in the scrotum and then the skin is sewn together on opposite sides, thus increasing the size. The lack of skin is perfectly covered (Shin et al., 2013).

The Epidemiology of Vaseline in and outside Prisons in Hungary

The self-injection of Vaseline is spread 80% among convicts or men with such connections; most of them are of Romany origin in Hungary, as well. From the 1900's onward the penis enlargement with petroleum jelly and paraffin oil as a drug appeared in Hungary, too. Several publications have appeared on the subject (Benedek, 1913; Tóth et al., 1984; Nyirády et al., 2008; Sejben et al., 2012). In 1984, Tóth et al. reported a multistage reconstructive surgery on a patient who had come forward due to a damage suffered as a result of paraffin oil.

In 2006, Kelemen and his colleagues presented the case of 16 patients, and showed the harmful consequences of the injection of petroleum jelly. In their work, they gave a detailed description of the surgical reconstruction options. Their patients reported that complications after the injection of petroleum jelly did not always occur. In case of early complications only major complaints made the patients see the doctor, they tried to keep the Vaseline injection secret. They tried to help themselves with cold compress and antibiotics or squeezing out the developed pus from their penis. Unfortunately, penis enlargements with petroleum jelly are carried out not only in prisons, but also in tattoo parlours (Kelemen et al., 2006).

Non-Invasive Methods of Penis Lengthening

Vacuum Device

The vacuum therapy is used to treat erectile dysfunction. Aghamir et al. examined the effect of vacuum therapy penis extender. In their study they involved healthy, sexually active men who were unhappy with their penis size. They treated their patients with the vacuum three times a week for 20 minutes in a 6 months long period. Although the vacuum treatment did not cause any significant increase of the penis, some patients had psychological satisfaction (Aghamir et al., 2006, Chung and Brock, 2013; Oderda and Gontero, 2011).

Penile Traction Therapy

The only effective non-surgical method of penis enlargement is the penile-extender device. The stretching of the penis with an extender device is also used for the treatment of Peyronie' disease and it is applied for magnifying the penis, as well. It is a relatively effective method and does not involve side effects. The patients tolerate it well and they are satisfied with the results. The device consists of a plastic ring, into which the penis is fixed; the glans is held by a silicone band. In between the two, the pulling is done by a dynamic metallic rod. The patients wear the tool for 4-9 hours a day for months, at least for 6 months. The volume and the time of the drawing will be gradually raised. The device exerts a progressive mechanical traction. The results hardly exceed 1.5 cm, but the patients are still satisfied, they tolerate the procedure easily and side effects hardly occur (Mondaini et al., 2002, Gontero et al., 2009; 2009; Nikoobakht et al., 2011).

Invasive Procedures to Increase the Penis

Extending with Rib Cartilage

The disassembly technique is used for the correction of congenital or acquired penile malformations (Perovic et al., 1998, 1999; Bajory et al., 2003, 2012; Király et al., 2008; Szalay et al., 2010) and by the man into woman gender reassignment surgeries (Perovic et al., 2000; Pajor et al., 2002). Perovic and Djordjevic used the disassembly technique in combination with rib cartilage implantation to increase the length of the penis. The surgery was done to patients who were dissatisfied with their penis size. Their erectile penis was originally 6-10 cm long. The surgical technique is the following: the penis is separated into anatomical units, sparing the neurovascular bundle and the urethra dissected from the corpora caversosas. Then the glans is also separated together with the neurovascular bundle. A gap arises between the glans and the corpora cavernosa, where the rib cartilage is inserted. The good blood supply of the subcutaneous tissue of the penis nourishes the rib cartilage so that it remains viable. The possible increase is limited by the urethral length and the flexibility of the neurovascular bundle. Perovic and colleagues were able to extend the penis with 2-4 cm, which the patients were satisfied with (Perovic and Djordjevic, 2000).

Phalloplasty Augmentation with Bilateral Saphena Grafts

Austoni and Cazzaniga could increase the volume of the corpus cavernosums with their surgical technology during erection. The diameter of the penis grows of 4.2 cm on average during erection. With this technique, they increased the tunica albuginea with the help of the saphena graft and through this the diameters of the corpus cavernosums grew. They made a sub-coronal incision on the penis and then separated the tissues from the Buck's fascia skeletonising it. They made a bilateral longitudinal incision on the Buck's fascia from the apex of the corpora cavernosa to the root of the penis, carefully sparing the neurovascular bundle. So as to measure the required size of the graft an artificial erection was established. The graft was obtained from the vein saphena. Then they incised the tunica albuginea and sewed the saphena patch onto it. They operated 39 patients with success and major postoperative complications did not occur (Austoni and Cazzaniga, 2002).

Suprapubic Dermatolipectomy with Liposuction

Many obese patients' penis disappears under the pubic skin fat or sag in the scrotum. The excess fat can be eliminated with plastic surgery (liposuction, lipectomy), thus the penis can seem larger (Alter et al., 2011; Alter, 2012).

Penile Suspensory Ligament Division

Chi-Ying Li and colleagues reported the results of 42 patients, where they achieved a penile augmentation by suspensory ligament division. The method itself can produce a 1.3-2 cm growth and the patients were partly satisfied. It was often accompanied by other penis enlargement methods. The function of the suspensory ligament is the stabilization of the penis, and by cutting it an optical gain can be achieved. During the surgery, the suspensory ligamentet was separated from the pubic bone. In the resulting gap silicone prosthesis was placed (small testicular prosthesis). 35% of the patients were satisfied with the results; almost 50% of them underwent another enlargement surgery later. Abnormal wound healing occurred by 5 patients in the postoperative period, which healed due to conservative therapy. Li et al. recommend the surgical methods of penis enlargement as a final solution only in patients with dysmorphophoby who understand that the achievable results are limited (Li et al., 2006).

The Aim of the Thesis

Our aim was to investigate a special case of self-harm of the penis. We studied the convicts' Vaseline self-injection, and our patients who had reconstructive surgery as a result of the suffered damage.

We explored the complications caused by self-injection of Vaseline, the motivation and the epidemiology in a sub-culture in Hungary. In addition, we explored the foreign objects inserted into the penis, the self-harm procedures and the typical populations and countries, where it has spread.

Methods

Our Cohort

At the Department of Urology University of Szeged there were 78 patients operated due to damage developed by self-injection of Vaseline between 2006 and 2012. A prospective study followed the patients. We assessed the circumstances of Vaseline self-injection; we asked about the amount of the injected Vaseline and the motivation. The patients were divided into three groups (A, B, C) based on the severity of complications and the types of the applied surgery.

The group A patients (N=40) had only aesthetic problems or acquired phimosis. They underwent circumcision or the local excision of Vaseline granulomas, followed by primary closure of the incision or use of a small pedicle scrotal island-flap (figure 6-7). This flap is practically a part of a pedicle scrotal flap previously described by Yachia (Yachia, 1986).

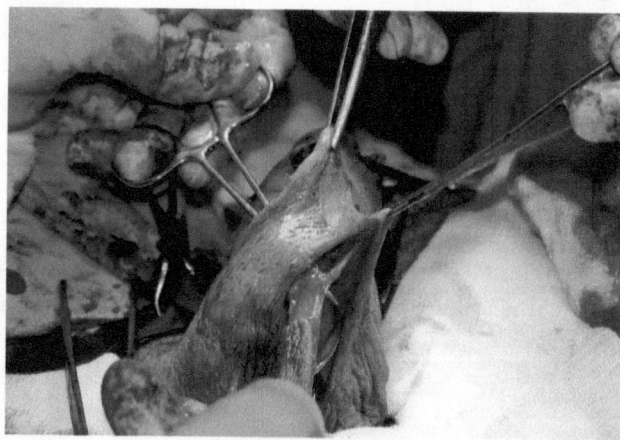

Figure 6 *The pedicle island flap is pulled up to the dorsal surface of the penis through a subcutaneous tunnel*

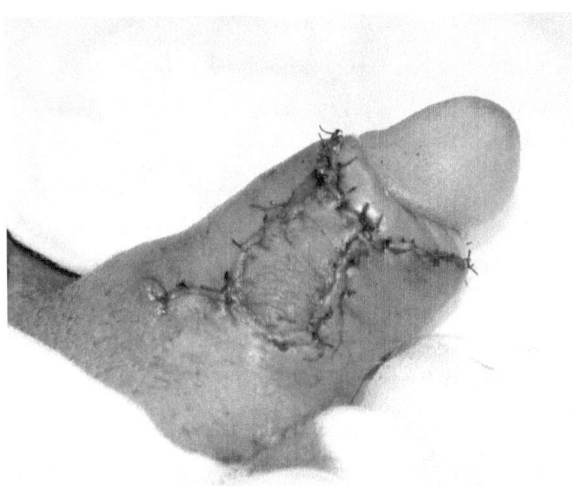

Figure 7 *The penile skin defect is replaced*

In group B (N=32), the patients had complications such as Vaseline granulomas, ulcers, and necrosis, which were localized on the penile skin and did not involve the scrotum. The affected penile skin was removed in these cases by removing the skin of the penis, performed from the distal to the proximal direction, over the cavernosal bodies, the dorsal neurovascular bundle and the urethra. Scrotal skin flaps were used to reconstruct the penile skin. In the initial cases (B/1, N=20), the penis without its skin layer was buried in a tunnel under the tunica dartos of the scrotum, as described in the previous literature (Yachia, 1986), where the tunnel is as long as the length of the stretched penis (figure 8).

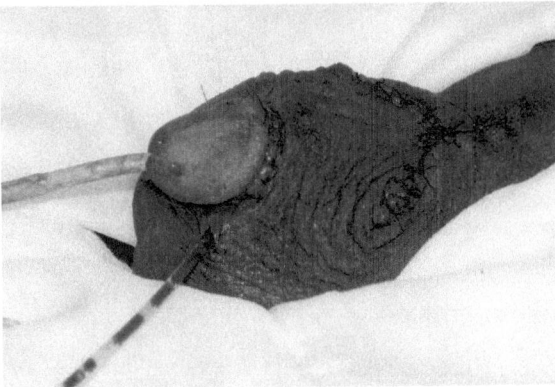

Figure 8 *The bare skinned penis is placed in a tunnel under the tunica dartos of the scrotum*

Three to five months after the surgery, when the new blood supply had formed, the penis was liberated, together with the surrounding scrotal skin. Tension-free closure of the wound was performed on the ventral part of the penis and the skin was closed above the testicles, too. When we had acquired more experience, a new modification of a previously described (Yachia, 1986) one-step reconstructive surgery (B/2, N=12) was developed. The penile skin was removed in the same manner. The dorsal side of the scrotum was opened along the raphe. The two scrotal-skin flaps were transluminated from the outside to the inside. This technique helps the surgeon visualize the anterior scrotal branches of the deep external pudendal artery and the posterior scrotal branches of the internal pudendal artery (figure 9). This kind of skin incision secures the anatomical structures without compromising the vascularity to minimize the postoperative necrosis of the edges of the skin. The bilateral scrotal flaps nourished by intact arterial branches were elevated and joined to the residual inner layer of the prepuce around the penile shaft and to each other on the dorsal surface of the penis with simple interrupted sutures.

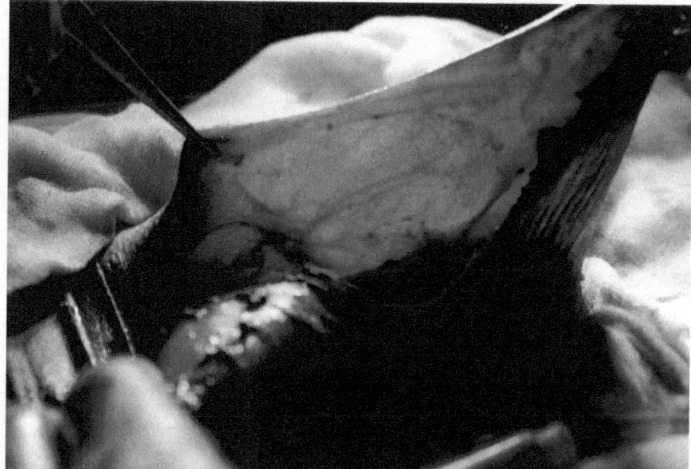

Figure 9 *The scrotal-skin flap is transluminated; the anterior scrotal branches of the deep external pudendal artery and the posterior scrotal branches of the internal pudendal artery are visualized*

The created skin flaps sometimes cannot cover the whole ventral-distal shaft of the penis in a tension-free manner and a triangular area remains naked. This area is covered by the inner layer of the prepuce, which is usually not affected by the Vaseline self-injection. This part of the prepuce is dissected dorsally, the bilateral inner layer of the prepuce is turned and pulled gently to a ventral position, and the flaps are sutured in the midline. If the patient has been circumcised previously or sufficient remaining intact prepuce is not available, a small split-thickness skin graft is used to cover this skin defect.

In group C (N=6), the patients exhibited Vaseline granulomas in both the penile and the scrotal skin. In these cases, the complete penile skin and a significant part of the scrotal skin were removed during the surgery. The penis was covered by the rest of the Vaseline-free scrotum. Since no scrotal skin remained available to cover the testicles, bilateral skin flaps from the femoral regions were elevated and trans-positioned medially to cover the testicles (Figure 10, 17). The patients were continuously monitored, and detailed physical examinations were made 1 and 3 months postoperatively. The patients were asked about the level of their satisfaction and their postsurgical sexual life. The duration of hospitalization was considered, and the removed skin was subjected to histological analysis.

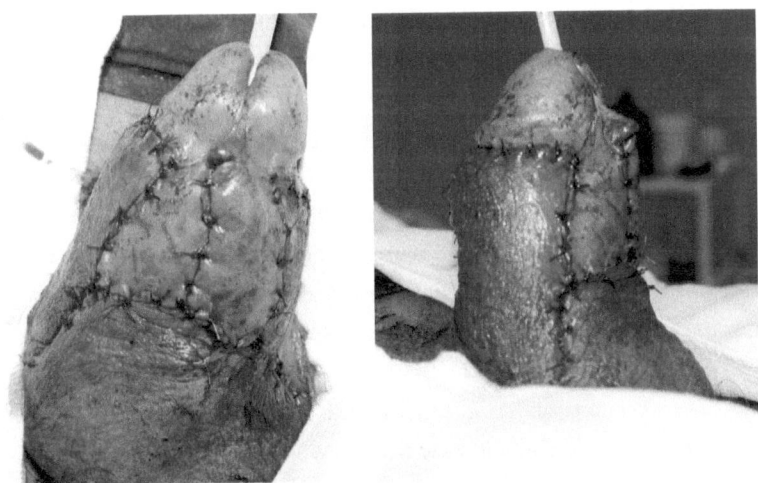

Figure 10 *Lateral and ventral aspects; the scrotal flaps are positioned and joined on the dorsal surface of the penis and the incision under the coronal sulcus is also closed. The bilateral prepuce flaps help to cover a triangular area on the distal part of the ventral surface. The proximal part of the ventral surface is covered by the pulled-up scrotum*

Questionnaire Survey in Prisons

This study involves a planned analysis of the incidence and morbidity of Vaseline self-injection among inmates of the six largest and strictest prisons in Hungary (located in Budapest, Szeged, Vác, Márianosztra, Sátoraljaujhely, and Sopronkőhida), through the use of a well-structured questionnaire. The results were analyzed statistically in order to assess the incidence of use of Vaseline self-injection, the motivations, the complications, the level of satisfaction, and the development of any sexual distress in this population. In 2010, with the permission of the Hungarian Prison Service Headquarters, informative lectures were given to the inmates in the above mentioned six Hungarian prisons, and a 17-point questionnaire was then distributed to 4,735 inmates. No inmates were excluded from the study. Those willing to participate gave their signed informed consent and completed the questionnaires independently. The questionnaires were collected anonymously, and returned to us by mail. A total of 1,905 inmates agreed to participate in this study and their questionnaires were analyzed statistically. The 17-item questionnaire, compiled by us, does not generate a numerical score. It had to contain easy questions due to the generally low level of education in this cohort. Its completion was anonymous and voluntary, without any engagement. It was designed to assess the incidence of use of Vaseline self-injection, the motivations, the complications, the level of satisfaction, the development of any sexual distress, and the appropriate function. The questionnaire asked about the duration of imprisonment, („What is the length of your sentence?") also asked about the level of satisfaction („Are you satisfied with the size of your penis?") and („Were you satisfied with your sexual life before imprisonment?"). It also enquired about the existence of any erectile dysfunction („Have you ever had any erectile dysfunction?"), if there were any details connected with Vaseline self-injections. („Has Vaseline ever been injected into your penis?"), („When was the Vaseline injected into your penis?"), („Approximately how much Vaseline was injected into your penis?"), („Who recommended you to inject Vaseline into your penis?"), („Do you have any problem with the injected Vaseline?"). We inquired about the levels of satisfaction before and after the self-injection („Were you satisfied with the size of your penis before the injection?"), („Were you satisfied with your sexual life before the injection?"), („Are you satisfied with the size of your penis now, after the injection?"), („Are you satisfied with the shape of your penis now?"). We also asked about the complications after the procedure („Have you had any erectile dysfunction since the injection?"), („Do you have any problem with the injected Vaseline, such as pain, tightening of the foreskin, wound/ulcer?"), („Have you regretted the Vaseline injection?"), ("Do you plan to ask for surgery to remove Vaseline from your penis?").

Dear Sir,
Vaseline self-injection into the skin is a quite common procedure in Hungarian prisons. Mild complications occur after the injection in 60% of the cases, and severe ones in 30%, which may need difficult reconstructive surgery to solve the problem. The more severe later complications are seen by doctors. Please help us with this study and the preventive work at the Department of Urology in Szeged, and complete the questionnaire. This is a voluntary questionnaire requiring no names, and the data are handled in total secrecy. There are no disadvantages of answering the questionnaire, but it can help many people in the future.

1. What is the length of your sentence? **less than 5 years   5–10 years   more than 10 years**
2. Have you ever had any erectile dysfunction?   Yes   No
3. Were you satisfied with your sexual life before imprisonment?   Yes   No
4. Has Vaseline ever been injected into your penis?   Yes   No
If NO, you need to answer only question 5. If YES, please continue answering with question 6.
5. Are you satisfied with the size of your penis?   Yes   No
6. When was the Vaseline injected into your penis?
0–6 months ago   6–24 months ago   more than 24 months ago
7. Who recommended this procedure?
No one   A sexual partner   A friend/relative   Prisoner   Stranger
8. Do you have any problem with the injected Vaseline?   Yes   No
9. If YES, what is the problem?
pain   tightening of the foreskin   wound/ulcer
10. Were you satisfied with the size of your penis before the injection?   Yes   No
11. Were you satisfied with your sexual life before the injection?   Yes   No
12. Are you satisfied with the size of your penis now, after the injection?   Yes   No
13. Are you satisfied with the shape of your penis now?   Yes   No
14. Have you had any erectile dysfunction since the injection?   Yes   No
15. Have you regretted the Vaseline injection?   Yes   No
16. If YES, do you plan to ask for surgery to remove the Vaseline from your penis? Yes   No
17. Approximately how much Vaseline was injected into your penis?
10 ml   20 ml   30 ml   40 ml
Thank you for your cooperation! After completing it, please put the questionnaire in the collecting box!

Figure 11 *Questionnaire*

Statistical Analysis

The statistical analysis was carried out by Statistica 7.0 (StatSoft Inc., Tulsa, OK, USA) software. We gave the descriptive statistics of the categorical scale measured data of the questionnaires in one-, two-or multi-way frequency tables and with the calculation of the appropriate percentage value. The statistical comparison of the frequency data were performed using the Pearson's Chi-square test and the Fisher's exact test.

We presented the data measured on a continuous scale and showing normal distribution by each group averages ± in the form of the mean standard error, and these data were evaluated by using vaccine analysis and Newman-Keuls post hoc test.

The deviations were always considered statistically significant in the case of $p<0.05$.

Results

Demographic Data

In Hungary 12,000 prisoners are being held. 17.6% of the convicts are 18-24 years old 16.8% are 25-29 years old, 36.3% are 30-39 years old, 21.2% are 40-49 years old and 8.2% are over 50 years of age. As for the level of education, 0.7% of the prisoners is illiterate, 64.8% left primary school, sometimes with only a few classes, and 19.6% finished vocational training, 13.6% finished secondary school and 1.3% graduated at college or university. As for their marital status: 54.6% of them are married or have a permanent sexual partner, 8.8% of them are divorced, 0.4% of them are widowed and 36.2% are single (table 1).

The inmates' data participating in our survey are identical to those of the total Hungarian data.

Age (years)	%
18-24	17,6
25-29	16,8
30-39	36,3
40-49	21,2
50-	8,2

Table 1 A: *The proportion of the Hungarian convicts categorized*

Education	%
Illiterate	0,7
Primary school	64,8
Vocational school	19,6
Secondary school	13,6
Bachelor or Master degree	1,3

Table 1 B: The *inmates' education by the length of their sentence*

Source: Almanac 2011 / 25th side
www.bvop.hu

Relationship	%
married	15,3
cohabit	39,3
single	36,2
divorced	8,8
widow	0,4

Table 1 C: *The inmates' marital status*

The Results of the Questionnaire Survey

4,735 (40.2%) of the inmates in the six prisons were involved in the study, 1,905 completed the questionnaire (in some cases, not all of the questions were answered). 37.5% (N=714) of the responders had received sentences of less than 5 years in prison, 34.8% (N=663) of them 5–10 years, and 16.8% (N=321) of them more than 10 years (table2).

Sentences (year)	0-5	5-10	10-
The proportion of the survey respondents (%)	37.5	34.8	16.8
Inmates (n=4735)	2368	1752	616
Completed the questionnaire (n=1905)	714	663	320
Completed the questionnaire (%)	30.2	37.8	52.0
Did not complete the questionnaire (%)	69.8	62.2	48.0

Table 2 *The proportion of the convicts categorized by the length of their sentence*

15.7% (N=299) of the responders admitted that they had injected Vaseline into their penis (figure12). 40.2% (N=119) of the Vaseline users, had received sentences of less than 5 years in prison, 38.5% (N = 114) of them 5–10 years, and 19.6% (N=58) of them more than 10 years. The proportion of those sentenced to more than 10 years was significantly smaller than that of those sentenced to a shorter period (p<0.05). The duration of the prison sentence did not influence the rate of Vaseline use (p=0.85). According to sporadic, verbal information from the inmates, the Vaseline injections are performed mostly among new inmates, during the first 3 months of their imprisonment. 299, 8.7% (N=26) of the responders had done it within the past 6 months, 15.4% (N=46) of them within the past 6–24 months, and 71.9% (N=215) more than 24 months previously (figure12).

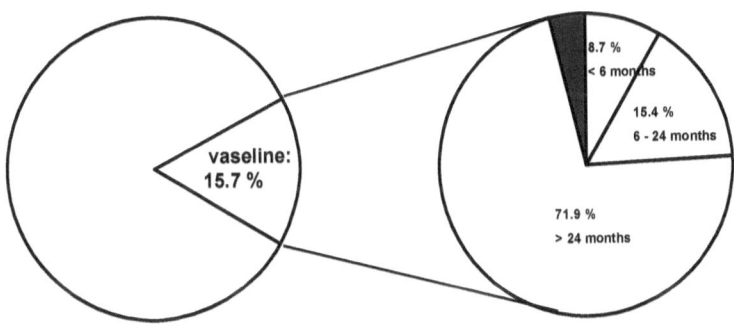

Figure 12 *15.7% (N=299) of the responders, admitted that they had injected Vaseline into their penis. 299, 8.7% (N=26) of the responders had done it within the past 6 months, 15.4% (N=46) of them within the past 6–24 months, and 71.9% (N=215) more than 24 months previously*

Vaseline injection was recommended by a fellow inmate in 44.1% (N=132) of the cases, a friend/relative in 20.7% (N=62), a stranger in 3.7% (N=11), a sexual partner in 9.7% (N=25), and no one in 18.1% (N=54) (table3).

Recommendation	%	N
Prisoner	44,10%	132
Friend/relative	20,70%	62
Stranger	3,70%	11
Nobody	18,10%	54
Sexual partner	9,70%	25
Total	96,30%	284

Table 3 *Different groups who recommended Vaseline self-injection to the respondent subjects*

Among the responders who had not performed Vaseline self-injection, only 7.6% (N=122) had suffered an erectile dysfunction, 77.9% (N=1246) of them were satisfied with their sexual life, and 75.1% (N=1202) of them were satisfied with the size of their penis.

21.1% (N=63) of the responders who had carried out Vaseline self-injection, had been dissatisfied with the original size of the penis and 19.0% (N=57) of them had been dissatisfied with their previous sexual life. There were no significant differences (p=0.47) between the two groups from these aspects after the Vaseline self-injection, 15.1% (N=45) of the subjects were dissatisfied with the size of the penis, 28.8% (N=86) were dissatisfied with the shape of the penis, and a de novo erectile dysfunction had developed in 21.4% (N=64) of them. These data differed significantly (p<0.001) from those relating the responders who had not injected Vaseline into their penis. In the group that had injected Vaseline into the penis, only a slight increase was later experienced concerning the level of satisfaction with the penile size (p=0.044) (figure 13).

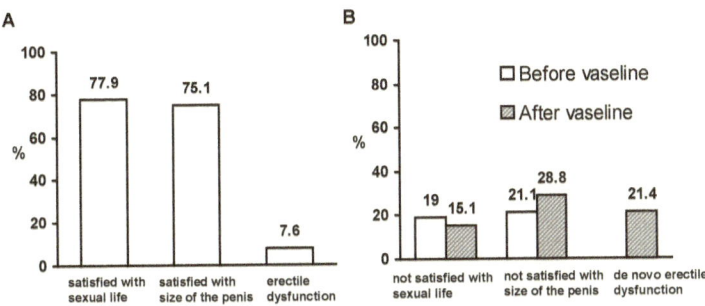

Figure 13 *The effect of injecting Vaseline on sexual life* **A:** *Those, who did not have Vaseline injected,* **B:** *Vaseline adopters. The Vaseline group 21.4% of the cases (N=64), de-novo erectile dysfunction developed. This value was significantly higher (p<0.001, Pearson's χ2-test between the observed and the expected frequencies) compared to the group with no Vaseline. Within the group using Vaseline there is only a marginal improvement in satisfaction related to penis size, after the injection of Vaseline. (p=0.044, Pearson's χ2-test)*

25.4% (N=76) of the responders who had self-injected Vaseline, admitted that there was subsequently some kind of abnormality in connection with their penis. In 31.6% (N=24) of them, phimosis had developed, 22.4% (N=17) had pain, and in 52.6% (N=40) a wound or ulcer had emerged (Figure 14).

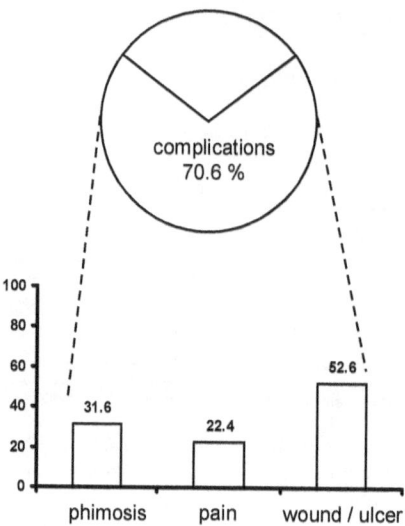

Figure 14 *Penile abnormalities in patients with complications of Vaseline self-injection*

29.1% (N=87) of the Vaseline users, regretted the self-injection, though the rate among those with complications was 53% (N=35). 72.4% (N=63), who regretted Vaseline self-injection, planned to participate in reconstructive surgery to remove the Vaseline.

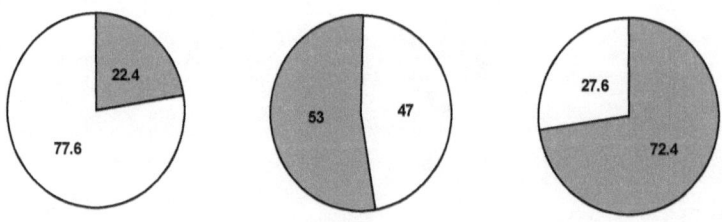

Figure 15 *22.4% of the Vaseline users regretted the self-injection; however, the rate who had complications was 53%; 72.4%, who regretted the Vaseline self-injection would undergo a reconstructive surgery to remove Vaseline*

The Results of the Penile Reconstruction

87.2% of the 78 patients operated on in our department were previous or present prison inmates. An additional 5.1% of the patients (N=4) admitted that they had not spent any time in prison, but the procedure had been recommended to them by a former inmate. Thus, 92.3% (N=72) of the Vaseline users had been in contact with prison life in some way. Sixty-eight (87.2%) of the patients had phimosis, and in 100% of them (N=78) thick, nodular Vaseline granulomas developed in the penis, ulcers occurred on the penile skin in 50% (N=39), and there was an extensive necrosis of the penile skin in 20.5% of the patients (N=16).

Group	N	Procedure
A (N=40)	32	Circumcision
	3	Circumcision + local excision
	3	Circumcision + local excision + scrotal island flap
	2	Local excision
B/1 (N=20)	20	Penis buried in the scrotum
B/2 (N=12)	7	One-step pedicled scrotal flaps
	4	One-step pedicled scrotal flaps + rotated prepuce
	1	One-step pedicled scrotal flaps + split-thickness skin graft
C (N=6)	6	Rotated scrotal flaps + transpositioned femoral skin flaps

Table 4 *Different types of procedures by groups*

In group A (N=40), local excision of the granuloma and/or circumcision were performed (Table 4). In most of these cases, the total removal of the Vaseline was not possible with these limited excisions. Thirty-one patients (77.5%) healed per primam and no postoperative complications occurred. In nine patients (22.5%), there were wound healing complications (probably caused by the residual Vaseline in the tissues), which needed local therapy and antibiotics. In group A, where the amount of Vaseline injected was 10–15 ml (Table 5), 100% of the patients were satisfied with the surgical and aesthetic results and were potent. The duration of hospitalization was 1–3 days (Table 5). In group B, where the amount of Vaseline injected into the penis was 20–40 ml (Table 5), a total removal of the penile skin was carried out because the self-injection affected the whole of the penile skin. In group B/1, where the penile shaft was buried beneath the dartos of the scrotum (Table 4), no complications were experienced in the early postoperative care following the first or second surgery, but in five cases (25%) postoperative marginal skin necrosis of the scrotal flap, placed on the penis, occurred 5–7 days after the second operation. In group B/2, postoperative marginal skin necrosis of the pedicle scrotal flaps developed in three cases (25%) in the first postoperative week. There were necrectomy, local therapy, and resuturing of the wound performed. There were areas, where a lack of skin healed per secundam. In one case (5%) in group B/1, the urethra near the coronal sulcus suffered an intra-operative injury during the removal of the Vaseline granuloma. The injury was treated with interrupted sutures, but these were not effective and a urethral fistula developed on the eighth postoperative day. During the second operation, the penis was separated from the scrotum, the fistula was closed, and the area above the fistula was covered by a split-thickness skin graft to avoid tension in this area. There were no complications after this procedure. In group B, 26 patients (81.2%) were satisfied with the surgical results, whereas six patients (18.7%) had aesthetic problems in connection with their penis, but none of them wanted additional surgery. None of them reported an erectile dysfunction. The duration of hospitalization was 4–28 days (Table 5). In group C, where the amount of Vaseline injected into the penis was 30–50 ml (Table 4), there were no complications of the trans-positioned scrotal skin flaps, but all of the femoral flaps covering the testicles shrank. This shrinkage caused only discomfort and mild complaints for the patients. All of the patients were satisfied with the surgical results (Figure16). The duration of hospitalization was 13–20 days (Table 5). Concerning the relationship between the amount of Vaseline and the duration of hospitalization, a one-way analysis of variance revealed significant differences among all the groups (Figure 16).

A: *The amounts of Vaseline injected (ml)*

Group	Means	N	Std.Dev.	Std.Err.	Minimum	Maximum
A	11.9	40	2.45	0.39	10	15
B	28.3	32	7.03	1.24	20	40
C	40.8	6	9.17	3.75	30	50

B: *Duration of hospitalization (days)*

Group	Means	N	Std.Dev.	Std.Err.	Minimum	Maximum
A	2.2	40	0.78	0.12	1	3
B	8.7	32	5.44	0.96	4	28
C	15.3	6	2.50	1.02	13	20

Table 5 *Descriptive statistics of patients in Group A-C*

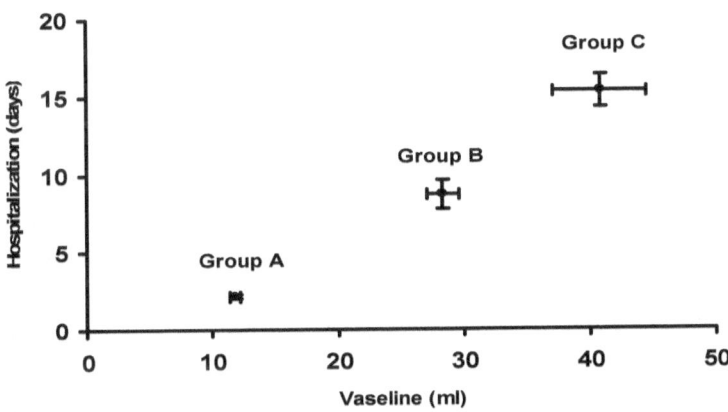

Figure 16 *Relationship between the mean amounts of Vaseline injected and mean duration of hospitalization in Groups A-C. Data are shown as mean ± std. error of mean. Groups were significantly different from each other regarding both parameter ($p<0.05$, ANOVA followed by Newman-Keuls post-hoc test)*

Three months after the surgery, 48 patients (61.5%) visited the outpatient department for control examinations. All of them were satisfied with their sexual life and none of them needed additional surgical correction (Figure 17). The histologic samples revealed chronic inflammation, a large number of foreign body giant cells, lymphocyte and hystiocyte infiltration with fibrosis, surface ulceration or chronic abscesses.

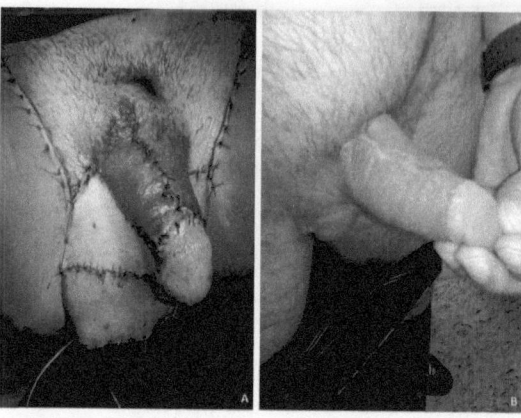

Figure 17 A: *The testicles are covered by the femoral transposition flaps* **B:** *Three months postoperatively. The femoral transposition flaps have slightly shrunk, but the patient experienced only discomfort.*

Discussion

The practice of placing foreign objects into the penis is as old as mankind, and in some subcultures it has the same popularity today. This practice however, brings the need of treating the defects caused by the foreign objects in the body imposing the burden on health care systems.

There is a growing trend of efforts for a bigger size of the penis these days. Many men underestimate his penis size and would like to extend it surgically. Unfortunately, the media also suggests that "bigger is better". Thus, men with a normal size penis also submit to an enlargement intervention. Penis enlargement surgery is only recommended in the case of real micro-penis. There are only few publications dealing with the indication of surgery and penis measurement techniques. The results differ, depending on the measurement technique and the measured population. The determination of a normal penis size is not unified either. It is questionable whether a few centimetre increase of the penis size can make the patient satisfied. Those, who are young, sexually active and healthy, have actually psychological dysfunction. In addition to surgical procedures, non-surgical and psychological therapies can be used, as well. The penis enlargement techniques may be only accepted if they cause a slight complication. Still there are only a few data and only a few patients who were followed in the long run. Nevertheless neither technique can be preferred (Vardi et al., 2008). Spyropoulos and colleagues developed a questionnaire that helped them to select the right patients for their penis enlargement surgery ("Augmentation Phalloplasty Patient Selection and Satisfaction Inventory/APPSSI"). Though their number of cases is small, the work calls attention to the fact that the surgical treatment of dysmorphophobia would be worthwhile and would need to standardize the pre-operative tests. The patients' sufficient motivation is critical to the successful surgeries. Their patients had undergone not only physical but also a psychological examination before the surgery. After the surgeries a few complications occurred, but their patients were satisfied with the results (Spyropoulos et al., 2005). Colombo and Casarico raise the ethical and psychological aspects of surgical penis enlargement. They recommend preoperative urological, psychosexual, psychological and psychiatric examination, where a multi-disciplinary team would work together (Colombo and Casarico, 2008).

According to Panfilov, the penis size is not a critical point for women. 90% of the nerve ends at the clitoris and 1 centimetre away from the introitus. The men want to meet the needs of their own not their partners'. They want to increase their self-confidence by turning to a plastic surgeon. They want to draw attention to the fact that the obtained results in centimetre a year after the surgery may even shrink. For penis filling autologous fat is recommend instead of foreign substances, which does not cause a foreign body reaction. For men who have larger than the normal penis size, the enlargement surgery is not recommended; rather the partner should be sent to a gynaecologist for vagina restriction (Panfilov, 2006).

Due to immigration, penile self-harm leads to public health problem not only in Eastern countries, but it spread in other parts of the world, as well. The patients do not see the physician in time, because of shame, or they remove the foreign body themselves. The complications are common, as the foreign object was implanted by themselves or to their fellow by laymen with no medical qualification and not in sterile conditions. It is common among convicts, sailors, labourers and soldiers.

The goal of implanting such materials are enhancing sexual pleasure, penis augmentation, bolding and decoration, masturbation, belonging to the same group, as well as symbolizing manliness or potency for some people (Stankov et al., 2009).

Lee et al. examined 26 cases in Korea, and 13 years later they could not found major problems only in 7 cases. They concluded that the complications developed, on average, approximately 18.5 months after the self-injection in the Asian population. Each of our patients reported that they had done it to emphasize their masculinity, but eventually pain and inflammation was the unfortunate outcome rather than the desired effect. Finally, the authors state that this self-destructive process afflicts mainly the men of lower social status with low education and there would be a great need for awareness-raising work (Lee et al., 1994).

Nyirády et al. reported on 16 European men who underwent corrective surgery, with accounts of the complications of the self-injection, the times between the self-injection procedures, and the development of complications, the reconstructive surgical techniques applied, and the overall results. In the European study, the authors created three groups (acute, sub acute, and chronic), examined the complications of the patients, and provided details of the histological characteristics of the abnormalities (Nyirády et al., 2008).

Moon at al. conducted a survey in a Korean prison in 2003. Each of the responders, a total of 357 men, increased the size of his penis with paraffin; of who 48.9% responded that a friend recommended the method. In 78% the procedure was not performed by a doctor. The reason why they embarked on it with 17.2%'s was the feeling of small penis size, with more than 32% was the concern of poor erectile function. But after the filling, only 33% of them got rid of their inferiority complex. 91% of respondents were dissatisfied with their penis afterwards, and 74% wanted to remove the material from their penis. Only 15.6% of them answered, that they did not have medical problem. The others suffered from various unpleasant complications (inflammation, necrosis, pain). By the psychological evaluation there were no answers that reflected pathological psychiatric differences. Finally, they called for the awareness and prevention work in this severely health damaging problem (Moon et al., 2003).

We determined the incidence of self-injection of Vaseline in Hungary's most affected population among prisoners in our representative study. The satisfaction with the original penis size and the sexual life was almost the same in the group of self-injectors prior to the intervention, similar to the group of non-adopters of petroleum jelly. Among the possible motives there are the false perception of their penis size, the erectile dysfunction, the following of the fellow prisoners' wrong example and the role of the size of the penis in the prison hierarchy, but the claim of sexual partners was not an important motivation for the intervention. Complications developed by a large number of Vaseline injectors.

The Vaseline appliers regretted their act and would like to remove the Vaseline surgically. The popularity of the intervention in this population can be attributed merely to the poor social conditions and ignorance, since the vast majority of Vaseline adopters are not satisfied with the aesthetic results. The severe cases often require complicated, multi-stage reconstructive surgery where we have to reckon with a non-negligible rate of complications. In Hungary the reconstructive surgery is not financed by the social security system, those who wish to heal cannot afford the surgery from their own resources; thus their treatment is delayed or cancelled.

In some sub-populations the incidence of Vaseline self-injection is higher than in the general population. The main motivation for the intervention is the fellow prisoners' bad example, so the information of these subpopulations about the harmfulness and ineffective nature of Vaseline self-injection is of essential importance. Our study of demonstrating the high incidence of complications of the petroleum jelly injection emphasizes the importance of prevention and education programs in order to improve the health and social status of the affected sub-population (Rosecker et al., 2011, 2012, 2013, 2013, 2013; Bajory et al., 2010, 2013).

Summary of New Scientific Results

1. A Survey of the Incidence of Vaseline Penis Augmentation in Hungarian Prisons

Our representative survey on the most affected population, the sentenced prisoners, showed a high incidence of Vaseline self-injection. The high incidence and the knowledge of complication rate revealed by our study can contribute to improve the health level of the affected sub-population. The injection of Vaseline is still a prevalent method for the enlargement of the penis. In some subpopulations the procedure is represented of 80% in prison, and spread among men with such connections, which is associated with severe complications. We performed a questionnaire survey based on the answers of 4735 convicts in the six largest and most rigorous prisons in Hungary. 1905 prisoners completed the questionnaire, the responses were statistically evaluated. 15.7% of the respondents admitted that Vaseline was injected into their penis. We learned that the main motivation for choosing it was the bad example of fellow prisoners. It can be clearly seen that among the injectors, even those who have not seen any doctor, there is a high occurrence of complications, and a clear correlation exists between the severity of complications and the amount of Vaseline injected. 29.1% of the Vaseline adopters regret the injection; the complication rate is 53% here. Among those who regretted 72.4% underwent surgical intervention to remove the Vaseline.

In this large, representative survey of the most affected population, we received a picture of a high incidence of self-injection. We can improve the health of this population concerned with prevention work, and proper information.

2. The elaboration of a new surgical technique for Vaseline penile reconstruction treatment

On our own patient population, which is the largest published patient population, the complications, surgical solutions, and reconstructive surgery innovation of reconstructive solutions of the Vaseline self-injection were reported. 78 patients were operated due to the developed damage of Vaseline self-injection between 2006 and 2012 at the Department of Urology in Szeged, and in 20 cases out of the 78 a multi-stage surgery was required.

We divided the patients into three groups (A, B, C) based on the severity of complications and the applied surgery types. Accordingly, they received stage-oriented care.

We listed the cases of aesthetic issue or causing phimosis in group A. These patients were treated by circumcision, local excision of the Vaseline granuloma and primary wound closure. In some cases, the defect was covered with a pedicle flap of the scrotal skin. In group B the lesions caused by Vaseline (granuloma, ulceration, necrosis) were localized under the skin of the penis, but the scrotal skin was intact. In these cases, the affected penile skin was removed, preserving the maximum part of the intact skin. The penis skin was released from distal to proximal direction, above the corpus cavernosum, the dorsal neurovascular bundle and the urethra. The skin replacement was performed with the scrotum skin. In our initial cases, we inserted the bare penis in a subcutaneous tunnel formed in the scrotum so that we calibrated the length of the subcutaneous tunnel to the stretched penile body length. After 3-5 months, when the collateral circulation established, we lifted the penis together with the scrotum skin on it. We made the incisions in the scrotum, thus we could close the skin on the ventral surface of the penis without tension. Then we also closed the remained scrotal skin over the testes. With the progress of our surgical practice, we performed the scrotal skin replacement in one session, using a new method. We removed the penile skin according to our current practice. Subsequently, we opened the dorsal surface of the scrotum along the raphe and brightly lighted skin flaps. With this method the arteria pudenda externa, supplying deep scrotal of the anterior branches of the artery and the back branches of the arteria pudenda interna, became well visible. Thus, we could save the form by sparing incisions of the skin, while preventing the postoperative necrosis. We collected the scrotal flaps belonging to the frontal supply area of scrotal branches with nodular stitches on the dorsal surface of the penis, and then under the glans we fixed them round, as well along the sulcus coronarius. The resulting flaps of skin usually cannot cover the ventral-distal portion of the penis in a triangular shape without stretching. We covered this area after the dorsal plate separation of the inner side of the mostly Vaseline intact foreskin, with turning the bilateral internal disk flap into ventral direction and covering it with merging in the central line.

We classified cases into group C where the Vaseline in-filtered the scrotal skin beside the penis skin. In these cases we had to remove not only the penis skin, but we had to resect a larger area of the scrotal skin. We carried out the penile skin replacement from the petrolatum intact scrotal skin in the manner already described, but there was no sufficient tissue to mask the testes. The skin covering of balls was carried out by the help of a plastic surgery method using the femoral flaps.

The treatment of complications caused by Vaseline is surgical. Conservative therapy does not result a permanent solution. In experienced hands the surgical reconstruction results healing, and the rate of complications is low.

References

Aghamir MK, Hosseini R, Alizadeh F. A vacuum device for penile elongation: fact or fiction?
BJU Int 2006; 97 (4): 777-8

Akkus E, Iscimen A, Tasli L et al. Paraffinoma and Ulcer of the External Genitalia After Self-injection of Vaseline. J Sex Med 2006; 3 (1): 170-2

Al-Ansari AA, Shamsodini A, Talib RA et al. Subcutaneous cod liver oil injection for penile augmentation: review of literature and report of eight cases. Urology 2010; 75 (5): 1181-4

Alei G, Letizia P, Ricottilli F et al. Original technique for penile girth augmentation through porcine dermal acellular grafts: results in a 69-patient series. J Sex Med 2012; 9 (7): 1945-53

Alter GJ, Salgado CJ, Chim H. Aesthetic of the male genitalia. Semin Plast Surg 2011; 25 (3): 189-95

Alter GJ. Pubic contouring after massive weight loss sin men and women: correction of hidden penis, mons ptosis, and labia majora enlargement. Plast Reconstr Surg 2012; 130 (4): 936-47

Anderson WR, Summerton DJ, Sharma DM et al., The Urologist's Guide to Genital Piercing. BJU Int 2003; 91 (3): 245-51

Angulo JC, García-Díez M, Martínez M. Phallic Decoration in Paleolithic Art: Genital Scarification, Piercing and Tattoos, J Urol 2011; 186 (6): 2498-503

Ardunio LJ., Sclerosing Lipogranuloma of Male Genitalia. J Urol 1959; 82 (1):155-61

Armstrong ML, Caliendo C, Roberts AE. Genital piercings: what is known and people with genital piercings tell us. Urol Nurs 2006; 26 (3): 173-9

Arthaud JB. Silicone-induced penile sclerosing lipogranuloma. J Urol 1973; 110 (2): 210

Austoni E, Guarneri A, Cazzaniga A. A new technique for augmentation phalloplasty: albugineal surgery with bilateral saphenous grafts--three years of experience. Eur Urol 2002; 42 (3): 245-53

Bajory Z, Pajor L, Perovic S, Borbély L. Veleszületett penis hiány pótlása. Magyar Urol 2003; 15 (4): 233-6

Bajory Z, Pajor L. Reconstructive surgery for vaseline-induced granulomas of the penile skin. J Sex Med 2010; 7(6): 443(P-11-001)

Bajory Z, Pajor L. A glans reszekciójának rekonstrukciós lehetőségei. Magyar Urol 2012; 24(3): 111

Bajory Z, Mohos G, Rosecker Á et al. Surgical Solutions for the Complications of the Vaseline Self-Injection of the Penis. J Sex Med 2013; 10 (4): 1170–7

Bayraktar N, Başar I. Penile Paraffinoma. Case Rep. Urol. 2012; (2012): 202840, 2

Bhat AL, Kumar A, Mathur SC et al. Penile Strangulation. Br J Urol 1991; (68): 618-21

Benedek L, Die paraffinome. Pester Med Chir Presse 1913; 49: 221

Blake-James BT, Hussain M, Peters JL., Genital foreign bodies: more than the eye can see. Eur J Emerg Med 2007; 14 (1): 53-5

Breyer NB, Shindel AW. Recreational urethral sounding is associated with high risk sexual behaviour and sexually transmitted infections. BJU Int 2012; 110 (5): 720–25

Brison D, Lamba S, Jafary A et al. Case report: urinary retention secondary to a foreign body in the male urethra. Emerg Radiol 2006; (13): 143-5

Bruno JJ, Senderoff DM, Fracchia JA et al. Reconstruction of penile wounds following complications of AlloDerm-based augmentation phalloplasty. Plast Reconstr Surg 2007; 119 (1): 1-4

Caliendo C. Self-reported characteristics of women and men with intimate body piercings. J Adv Nurs 2005; 49 (5), 474-84

Carlson HE. Sclerosing lipogranuloma of the penis and scrotum. J Urol 1968; 100 (5): 656-8

Carroll ST, Riffenburgh RH, Roberts TA et al. Tattoos and body piercings as indicators of adolescent risk-taking behaviors. Pediatrics 2002; 109 (6): 1021-7

Chung E, Brock G. Penile traction therapy and Peyronie's disease: a state of art review of the current literature. Ther Adv Urol 2013; 5 (1): 59-65

Cohen EL, Kim SW. Subcutaneous artificial penile nodules. J Urol 1982; 127 (1): 135

Cohen JL, Keoleian CM, Krull EA. Penile paraffinoma: self-injection with mineral oil. J Am Acad Dermatol 2001;45 (6): 222-4

Colombo F, Casarico A: Penile enlargement. Curr Opin Urol 2008; 18 (6): 583-8

Djajakusumah TS, Meheus A. Artificial nodules of the penis: case report of an Indonesian man. Sex Transm Dis 2000; 27 (3): 152-3

Edlin RS, Aaronson DS, Wu AK et al. Squamous cell carcinoma at the site of a Prince Albert's piercing. J Sex Med. 2010; 7 (6): 2280-3

Ekelius L, Fohlman J, Kalin M. The risk of severe complications of body piercing should not be underestimated. Lakartidningen 2005;102 (37): 2560-2

Fischer N, Hauser S, Brede O et al. Implantation of artificial penile nodules--a review of literature. J Sex Med 2010; 7 (11): 3565-71

Gan W, Yang R, Ji C et al. Case Report: Successful Remove of a Metal Axletree Causing Penile Strangulation in a 19-Year-Old Male by Degloving Operation. Case Rep Med 2012; 2012: 532358.

Gauthier M. Observation d'un étranglemant des testicules et de la verge, occasionné par le passage d'un briquet. J Med Chir Pharmacol (Paris) 1755; (3): 358

Glicenstein J. Les Premiers « fillers », vaseline et paraffine. Du miracle à la catastrophe. The first « fillers », vaseline and paraffin. From miracle to disaster Annales de chirurgie plastique et esthétique 2007; 52 (2):157-161

Gokhale R, Hernon M, Ghosh A. Genital piercing and sexually transmitted infections. Sex Transm Infect 2001; 77 (5): 393–4

Gold MA, Schorzmann CM, Murray PJ et al. Body piercing practices and attitudes among urban adolescents. J Adolesc Health 2005; 36 (4): 352.e 17-24

Gontero P, Di Marco M, Giubilei G et al. A pilot phase-II prospective study to test the 'efficacy' and tolerability of a penile-extender device in the treatment of 'short penis'. BJU Int 2009; 103 (6): 793-7

Gontero P, Di Marco M, Giubilei G et al. Use of penile extender device int he treatment of penile curvature as a result of Peyronie's disease. Results of a phase II prospective study. J Sex Med 2009; 6 (2): 558-66

Griffith J, Horowitz D. Penile nodules in the penal system. Cutis 2012; 89 (5): 237-9

Gürdal M, Karaman MI. An Usual Case of Penile Augmentation: Subcutaneous stone implantation. Urology 2002; 59 (3): 445

Holbrook J, Minocha J, Laumann A. Body Piercing Complications and Preevention of Health Risks. Am J Clin Dermatol 2012; 13 (1): 1-17

Hounsfield V, Davies SC. Genital piercing in association with gonorrhoea, chlamydia and warts. Int J STD AIDS 2008; 19 (7): 499-500

Hsu TH. Artificial penile nodules. Urology 2004; 63 (1): 174

Hudak SJ, McGeady J, Shindel AW et al. Subcutaneous penile insertion of domino fragments by incarcerated males in southwest United States prisons: a report of three cases. J Sex Med 2012; 9 (2): 632-4

Hull TH, Budiharsana M. Male Circumcision and penis enhancement in Southeast Asia: Matters of pain and pleasure. Reprod Health Matters 2001; 9 (18): 60-7

Hwang EC, Kim JS, Jung SI, et al. Delayed diagnosis of an intraurethral foreign body causing urosepsis and penile necrosis. Korean J Urol 2010; 51 (2): 149-51

Imbert E, Milpied B, Jouary T et al. Penile swelling and ulceration. Acta Derm Venereol 2010; 90 (1): 81-2

Ivanovski O, Stankov O, Kuzmanoski M et al. Penile strangulation: two case reports and review of the literature. J Sex Med 2007; 4 (6): 1775-80

Jaiswal AK. An unusual foreign body is the preputial sac. Genitourin Med 1992; 68(5): 334-5

Jindarak S, Angspatt A, Loyvirat R et al. Bilateral scrotal flaps: a skin restoration for penile paraffinoma. J Med Assoc Thai 2005; 88 (4): 70-3

Józsa L. Az emberi test mesterséges módosítása (deformálása). Orv Hetil 2011; 152 (36): 1462-5

Jung G., Park SJ., Seo J. A novel penoplasty technique for severe paraffinoma: modified bilateral scrotal flaps. J Urol 2012; 187 (4): 40

Kaatz M, Elsner P, Bauer A. Body-modifying concepts and dermatologic problems: tattooing and piercing. Clin Dermatol 2008; 26 (1): 35-44

Kadouch JA, van Rozelaar L, Kanhai RJC, et al. Complications of penis or scrotum Enlargement Due to Injections with Permanent Filling Substances. Dermatol Surg 2012;38 (7 Pt 2): 1244-50

Kang DH, Chung JH, Kim YJ, et al. Efficacy and Safety of Penile Girth Enhancement by Autologus Fat Injection for Patients with Thin Penises. Aesthetic Plast Surg 2012; 36 (4): 813-8

Kang SP, Chakravarti A, Amer K. Help of the fire brigade in a case of a strangulated penis. Ann R Coll Surg Engl. 2002; 84(5): 369-70

Karakan T, Ersoy E, Hasçiçek M et al. Injection of vaseline under penis skin for the purpose of penis augmentation. Case Rep Urol 2012; (2012): 510612

Katz DJ, Chin W, Appu S et al. Novel Extraction Technique to Remove a Penile Constriction Device. J Sex Med 2012; (9): 937-40

Kelemen Z, Nyirády P, Bánfi G et al. A hímvessző vastagítása vazelinnel – következmények és azok ellátása. Magyar Urol 2006; 18 (1): 16-27

Kelemen Z, Nyirády P, Németh Z et al. Hímvesszőre húzott fémgyűrű súlyos következményei. Magyar Urol 2005; 17 (4): 229–33

Kim JJ, Kwak TI, Jeon BG et al. Human glans penis augmentation using injectable hyaluronic acid gel. Int J Impot Res 2003; 15 (6): 439-43

Király I, Deák G, Őry-Tóth Cs et al. Hímvesszőt leszorító gyűrű sürgős eltávolítása gyors fémvágó körfűrésszel a merevedés megőrzése érdekében. Magyar Urol 2007; 19 (4): 204-6

Király I, Pajor L, Perovic S et al. Közösülési képesség helyreállítása húgycsőhiányos epispadiasisban. Magyar Urol 2008; 20 (2): 85-8

Ko CJ, Sarantopoulos G, Bhuta S et al. Scalp paraffinoma underlying squamous cell carcinoma. Arch Pathol Lab Med 2004; 128(10): 1171-2

Kokkonouzis I, Antoniou G, Droulias A. Penis deformity after intra-urethral liqud paraffin administration in a young male: a case report. Cases Journal 2008; (1): 223

Lamba S, Patel NN, Scott SR. Penile incaceration secondary to an S-Shaped lead pipe: removal with dremel moto-tool. J Emerg Med 2012; 42 (6): 659-61

Lee T, Choi HR, Lee YT et al. Paraffinoma of the penis. Yonsei Medical Journal 1994; 35 (3): 344-8

Levy G, Mercer D, Amosi D et al. Self-implanted artifical nodules: a computed tomography mimic of penile pathology. Acta Radiol 2008; 49 (2): 236-8

Li C, Kayes O, Kell PD et al. Penile suspensory ligament division for penile augmentation: indications and results. Eur Urol 2006; 49 (4): 729-33

Lim KB, Seow CS, Tulip T et al. Artificial penile nodules: case reports. Genitourin Med 1986; 62 (2): 123-5

Magrill D, Shabbir M, Belal M et al. Penile silicone pseudocarcinomatous epithelial hyperplasia; why bigger is not always better. British Journal of Medical and Surgical Urology 2008; (1): 139-41

Manny T, Pettus J, Hemal A et al. Penile sclerosing lipogranulomas and disfigurement from use of "1Super Extenze" among Laotian immigrants. J Sex Med 2011; 8 (12): 3505-10

Mastromichalis M, Sackman D, Cheval MJ Urethral foreign body insertion for secondary gain in the incarcerated population. Can J Urol 2011; 18 (5): 5916-7

May JA, Pickering PP. Paraffinoma of the penis. Calif Med 1956; 85 (1): 42–4

Micheels P, Saint Hillier S, Elias B et al. Hyaluronan and the "mushroom" technique: an assessment of hyaluronan injections into the glans. Dermatol Surg 2012; 38 (2): 1-7.

Mitterberger M, Peschel R, Frauscher F et al. Allen key completely in male urethra: a case report. Cases journal 2009; (2): 7408

Molnár I, Szőke D. Penis-strangulatio ritka esete. Magyar Sebészet 1973; (26): 335-6

Mondaini M, Ponchietti R, Gontero P et al. Penile length is normal in most men seeking penile lengthening procedures. Int J Impot Res 2002; 14 (4): 283-6

Moon DG, Kwak TI, Cho HY et al. Augmentation of glas penis using injectable hyaluronic acid gel. Int J Impot Res 2003; 15 (6): 456-60

Moon DG, Yoo JW, Bae JH et al. Sexual function and psychological characteristics of penile paraffinoma. Asian J Androl 2003; 5 (3): 191-4

Mooreville., Meller M. Penile incarceration with barbell retaining ring. J Urol 2001; 166(2): 618

Nakamura M, Sakurai T, Yoshida K et al. Sclerosing lipogranuloma of the penis: chemical analysis of lipid from the lesional tissue. J Urol 1985; 133 (6): 1046-8

Narins RS, Beer K. Liquid injectable silicone: a review of its history, immunology, technical considerations, complications, and otential. Plast Reconstr Surg 2006; 118 (3): 77-84

Nelius T, Armstrong ML, Rinard K et al. Genital piercings: diagnostic and therapeutic implications for urologists. Urology 2011;78(5): 998-1007

Nikoobakht M, Shahnazari A, Rezaeidanesh M et al. Effect of penile-extender device in increasing penile size in men with shortened penis: preliminary results. J Sex Med 2011; 8 (11): 3188-92

Noh J, Kang TW, Heo T et al. Penile strangulation treated with the modified string method. Urology 2004; 64 (3): 591

Nyirády P, Kelemen Z, Kiss A et al. Treatment and outcome of vaseline-induced sclerosing lipogranuloma of the penis. Urology 2008; 71 (6): 1132-7

Oderda M, Gontero P. Non-invasive methods of penile lengthening: fact or fiction? BJU Int 2011; 107 (8): 1278-82

van Ophoven A, de Kernion JB. Clinical management of foreign bodies of the genitourinary tract. J Urol 2000; 164 (2): 274-87

Panfilov DE. Augmentative Phalloplasty. Aesthetic Plast Surg 2006; 30 (2): 183-97

Pajor L, Bajory Z, Deák G. Férfi-nő irányú transzszexuális műtét két esetben. Magyar Urol 2002; 14 (1): 11-4.

Pannek J, Martin W. Penile entrapment in a plastic bottle. J Urol. 2003; 170 (6 Pt 1): 2385

Parnitvitidkun S. Two-Staged Scrotal Tunnel Flap Repair: Treatment of Self-administered Penile Injection. Siriraj Med J 2007; 59 (3): 119-21

Pastides P, Lunawat R, Miller R et al. Use of the Dundee technique to relieve penile strangulation. British Journal of Medical and Surgical Urology 2011; (4): 213-15

Peay J, Smithson J, Nelson J et al. Safe emergency department removal of a hardened steel penile constriction ring. J Emerg Med 2009; 37 (3): 287-89

Pehlivanov G, Kavaklieva S, Kazandjieva J et al. Foreign-body granuloma of the penis is sexually active individuals (penile paraffinoma). J Eur Acad Dermatol Venereol 2008; 22 (7): 845-51

Perovic SV, Vukadinovic V, Djordjevic ML et al. The penile disassembly technique in hypospadiasis repair. Br J Urol 1998; 81 (3): 479-87

Perovic SV, Stanojevic DS, Djordjevic ML. Vaginoplasty in male transsexuals using penile skin and urethral flap. BJU Int 2000; 86 (7): 843-50.

Perovic SV, Vukadinovic V, Djordjevic ML et al. Penile disassembly technique for epispadiasis repair: variants of technique. J Urol. 1999; 162 (3 Pt 2): 1181-4

Perovic SV, Byun JS, Scheplev P et al. New perspectives of penile echancement surgery: tissue engineering with biodegradable scaffolds. Eur Urol 2006; 49 (1): 139-47

Perovic SV, Djordjevic ML. Penile lengthening. BJU Int 2000; 86 (9): 1028-33

Rinard K, Nelius T, Hogan L et al. Cross-sectional study examining four types of male penile and urethral „play". Urology 2010; 76 (6): 1326-33

Rosecker Á, Bajory Z, Pajor L. A vazelin öninjekciózás incidenciája és szövődményrátája. Magyar Urol 2011; 23 (3): 138

Rosecker Á, Pajor L, Bajory Z. A vazelin pénisz incidenciája és morbiditása. Magyar Urol 2012; 24 (2): 58-63

Rosecker Á, Bordás N, Pajor L et al. Hungarian „Jailhouse Rock": incidence and morbidity of vaseline self-injection of the penis. J Sex Med 2013; 10(2): 509-15

Rosecker Á, Pajor L, Bajory Z. Vazelin pénisz végleges gyógyítása többlépcsős műtéttel. Magyar Urol 2013; 25 (3): 145

Rosecker Á, Pajor L, Bajory Z. From body piercing to vaseline. Self-injuries of the penis. Eur Urol Today, 2013; 25(3): 26

Rosenberg E, Romanowsky I, Asali M et al. Tree cases of penile paraffinoma: a conservative approach. Urology 2007; 70 (2): 372.e9-10

Salles AG, Lotierzo PH, Gemperli R et al. Complications after polymethylmethacrylate injections: report of 32 cases. Plast Reconstr Surg 2008; 121 (5):1811-20

Santos P, Chaveiro A, Nunes G et al. Penile paraffinoma. J Eur Acad Dermatol Venereol 2003; 17 (5): 583-4

Santucci RA, Zehring RD, McClure D. Petroleum jelly lipogranuloma of the penis treated with excision and native skin coverage. Urology 2000; 56 (2): 331

Scholten E. An unusual complication of penile piercing. Br J Plast Surg 2005; 58 (4): 577-81

Schultheiss D, Mattelaer JJ and Hodges FM. Preputial infibulation: from ancient medicine to modern genital piercing. BJU Int 2003; 92 (7): 758-63

Sejben I, Rácz A, Svébis M et al. Petroleum jelly-induced penile paraffinoma with inguinal lymphadenitis mimicking incarcerated inguinal hernia. Can Urol Assoc J 2012; 6 (4): 137-9

Shaeer O, Shaeer K. Delayed complications of gel injection for penile girth augmentation. J Sex Med 2009; 6 (7): 2072-8

Shamsodini A, Al-Ansari AA, Talib RA et al. Complications of penile augmentation by use of nonmedical industrial silicone. J Sex Med 2012; 9 (12): 3279-83

Shin YS, Zhao C, Park JK. New reconstructive surgery for penile paraffinoma to prevent necrosis of ventral penile skin. Urology 2013; 81 (2): 437-41

Silberstein J, Downs T, Goldstein I. Penile injection with silicone: case report and review of the literature. J Sex Med 2008; 5 (9): 2231-7

Silberstein J, Grabowski J, Lakin C et al. Penile constriction devices: case report, review of the literature, and recommendations for extrication. J Sex Med 2008; 5 (7): 1747-57

Sinopidis X, Alexopoulos V, Panagidis A et al. Internet Impact on the Insertion of Genitourinary Tract Foreign Bodies in Childhood. Case Rep Pediatr 2012; (2012): 102156

Skegg K, Nada-Raja S, Paul C et al. Body piercing, personality, and sexual behavior. Arch Sex Behav 2007; 36 (1): 47-54

Solomon MP, Komlo C, De Frain M. Allograft materials in phalloplasty, a comparative analysis. Ann Plast Surg 2013; 71 (3): 297-9

Soyer HP, Petritsch P, Glavanovitz P et al. Sclerosing lipogranuloma (paraffin-induced granuloma) of the penis with a clinical picture of carcinoma. Hautarzt 1988; 39 (3): 174-6

Spyropoulos E, Christofordis C, Borousas D et al. Augmentation phalloplasty surgery for penile dysmorphophobia in young adults: considerations regarding patient selection, outcome evaluation and techniques applied. Eur Urol 2005; 48 (1): 121-7

Stankov O, Ivanovski O, Popov Z. Artificial penile bodies-from kama sutra to modern times. J Sex Med 2009; 6 (6): 1543-8

Steffens J, Kosharskyy B, Hiebl R et al. Paraffinoma of the extrenal genitalia after auto-injection of vaseline. Eur Urol 2000; 38 (6): 778-81

Sukkarieh T, Smaldone M, Shah B. Multiple foreign bodies in the anterior and posterior urethra. Int Braz J Urol 2004; 30 (3): 219-20.

Szalay I, Bordás N, Bajory Z, Pajor L. Esztétikus glans csonkolás péniszrák esetén. Magyar Urol 2010; 22 (1): 6-12

Torricelli FCM, de Andrade EM, Marchini GS et al. Penile enlargement with methacrylate injection: is it safe? Sao Paulo Med J 2013; 131 (1): 54-8

Tóth M, Kántor M, Meluzsin J et al. Paraffinolaj penis bőre alá történő injiciálásának esete. Urol Nephrol Szle 1984; 11 (2): 112-3

Trockman BA, Berman CJ, Sendelbach K et al. Complication of penile injection of autologous fat. J Urol 1994; 151 (2): 429-30

Vardi Y, Harshai Y, Gil T et al. A Critical Analysis of Penile Enhancement Procedures for Patients with Normal Penile Size: Surgical Techniques, Success, and Complications. Eur Urol 2008; 54 (5): 1042-50

Walsh P, Moustafa M. Retention of urethrovesical foreign bodies: case report and literature review. J Emerg Med 2000; 19 (3): 241-3

Wessell HS, Lue TF, McAninch JW. Penile length in the flaccid and erect states: Guidelines for penile augmentation. J Urol 1996; 156 (3): 995-7

Wiwanitkit W. Penile injection of foreign bodies in eight Thai patients. Sex Transm Infect 2004; 80 (6): 546

Wylie KR, Eardley I. Penile size and the 'small penis syndrome'. BJU Int 2007; 99 (6): 1449-55

Yachia D. A new one-stage pedicled scrotal skin graft urethroplasty. J Urol 1986; 136 (3): 589–92

Yacobi Y, Tsivian A, Grinberg R et al. Short-term results of incremental penile girth enhancement using liquid injectable silicone: words of praise for a change. Asian J Androl 2007; 9(3): 408-13

Zickerman PM, Ratanawong C. Penile oleogranuloma among Wisconsin Hmong. WMJ 2007; 106 (5): 270-4

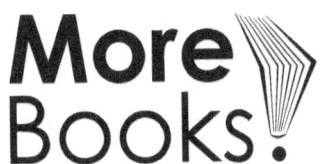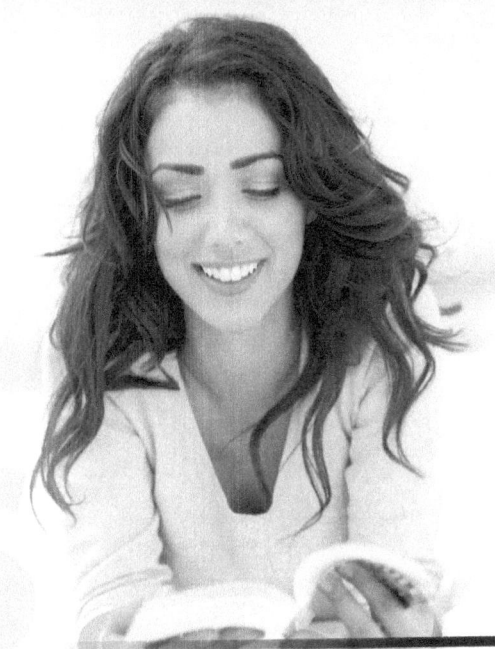

i want morebooks!

Buy your books fast and straightforward online - at one of world's fastest growing online book stores! Environmentally sound due to Print-on-Demand technologies.

Buy your books online at
www.get-morebooks.com

Kaufen Sie Ihre Bücher schnell und unkompliziert online – auf einer der am schnellsten wachsenden Buchhandelsplattformen weltweit! Dank Print-On-Demand umwelt- und ressourcenschonend produziert.

Bücher schneller online kaufen
www.morebooks.de

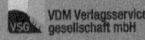 VDM Verlagsservicegesellschaft mbH
Heinrich-Böcking-Str. 6-8   Telefon: +49 681 3720 174   info@vdm-vsg.de
D - 66121 Saarbrücken   Telefax: +49 681 3720 1749   www.vdm-vsg.de

www.ingramcontent.com/pod-product-compliance
Lightning Source LLC
Chambersburg PA
CBHW031545210526
45464CB00003B/1162

* 9 7 8 3 6 5 9 5 3 2 9 5 5 *